The
ROAD
to
HEALING

The ROAD to HEALING

Turning Yesterday's Pain into the Stepping Stones that Lead to Your Destiny

JANNA VALENCIA

ROAD TO HEALING

Turning Yesterday's Pain into the Stepping Stones that Lead to Your Destiny

Janna Valencia

All scripture references are from the Holy Bible, New International Version unless otherwise indicated.

First edition: June 2016: 9780997460605

Oxford King Publishers
207 E. Brazos Street
Palestine, TX 75801

ISBN: 978-0-9974606-0-5 (softcover)

ISBN: 978-0-9974606-1-2 (ebook)

Contents

Acknowledgments

Janice Burris, my mom and mentor

Melinda Dowden, who had the faith
to show me the love of Jesus

Debbie Harvey McKinney, whose unconditional love and friendship inspired me to
grow even through the hard times

Tom Ziglar, Julie Ziglar Norman, Cindy
Ziglar Oates and the staff at Ziglar, Inc., who
inspired me to find my purpose in life

Howard Partridge and the entire staff at
Phenomenal Products, whose continual love and
support have helped me achieve my dreams

Michelle Prince for the encouragement
and inspiration to publish my book

FOREWORD

Julie Ziglar

Some people stand out, and Janna Valencia is one of them. Her confidence is immediately recognizable and her creativity is undeniable, but it is her love for others that stems from her faith in Jesus Christ that attracts everyone to her.

When I read Janna's book, *The Road to Healing: Releasing Your Pain and Finding Your True Purpose*, what moved me most was her utter transparency. God has called her to be honestly frank about her past failures so that she can encourage those who still struggle in their journey to a better way of life.

Janna's own victory over drug and alcohol addiction and her recovery from verbal, mental and physical abuse has equipped her to show others the path to the life they will love to live.

I was drawn into her life story immediately and was touched as I read how she accepted responsibility for her choices. Ultimately, Janna came to understand where wrong thinking had led her down a self-destructive path as she looked for love and acceptance where it could not be found.

I know you will be drawn into her story of the freedom healing gives and how she found her true purpose in life. I believe her journey can help you discover where your healing AND your true purpose in life can be found.

Julie Ziglar Norman, Author, Keynote Speaker, Life Coach and Founder of Ziglar Women

INTRODUCTION

It is my great honor to write this book and an even greater honor that you have decided to read it. May it bless your life in every way.

I have spent my entire life learning what I should *not* do, and this knowledge has given me the ability to share with you what I have learned. I was once ashamed of my past and the things I experienced. I did not want anyone to know I had failed multiple times in marriage or that I was addicted to drugs. I did not want anyone to know I permitted my husband to abuse me or that I was so insecure I was willing to participate in illegal and immoral acts in order to feel significant and loved.

I made many mistakes, each of which has been added to my "book of life." What you will find in this book is an accounting of these experiences and how they taught me to reach past my circumstances to find something meaningful and fulfilling for my future. They taught me how to find my purpose when there was no one else to help me.

I did not start out with some incredible intelligence or an abundance of money. I grew up in an average family with a brother and two sisters. Both of my parents worked. We lived in a quiet country town and I grew up on the family farm. I was an average student in high school. I did not get a college degree, but learned my skills from experience, so when I say, "If I can do it, you can do it," I sincerely mean it. I am no different from you. We both have the ability to be, do, or have whatever we desire, if we are willing apply a few simple concepts to make it a reality.

Today, I am an entrepreneur and successful business owner. I have received my certification as a Ziglar Legacy speaker and trainer, and as a Robbins Madanes Coach. Both of these certifications grew out of my desire to realize my true purpose and share it with the world in the most effective way possible.

My time and business are dedicated to helping others in many areas of their personal and professional lives. It does not matter who you are, where you have been, or what you have been through, I know you can find your way out of any difficulties and achieve your destiny.

I have built businesses from the ground up and experienced both success and failure. The successes far outweigh the failures, but even the failures have been great learning experiences that have helped me become more knowledgeable. The personal experiences I have been through are tools for learning anyone can apply.

The common element for all of us is that we have the same needs, even though our lives might have been very different. As we go through life, our needs are met, or not met, through the things we do and the people who are in our lives. When these elements change or become unhealthy and our needs are no longer being met, we begin looking in other places. When we are able to associate meeting a need with a person, place, or thing – and we believe we have found a way to fulfill our need, we will do and say things that are based on this association. This is not a permanent solution to meeting the need that is temporarily being met. Over the course of time, this time frame will vary widely, we become discontent because our association and actions were not permanent. To find a permanent solution and stop living in a temporary state of fulfillment, we must find new ways of getting our needs met.

You may not have had the kinds of experiences in your life that I have, or maybe you have had more. I know it is difficult to believe that someone else could understand what you are going through, but if you are willing to continue reading you will come to understand that the information in this book can help you find the answers you need to overcome your pain and begin to live again. It does not matter what the level of your experience was, or is. You *can* overcome adversity by taking a series of small steps that will help you find direction in your life. I understand that you are lost and hurting, and you find it hard to see "the light at the end of the tunnel," but I assure you that if you walk with me through the process in this book, you will find or regain your true purpose.

While writing this book, I questioned myself as to why I would want to reveal to the world that I had these problems in my past. Everyone knew me as a strong, determined, successful person who had it all together. The answers were resounding.

The first answer came from my Lord, God. In the Bible, we are instructed to go out into the world and share the Good News.

The second answer came from within me: My purpose is to help others be, do, and have more in their lives. My life is a living, breathing example of how you can overcome your past, find your true purpose, and ultimately reach your destiny.

Some of you reading this book might not have any idea why you feel there is no purpose to your life, or ask yourself why you feel unloved. It's okay. During this process, we will search for these reasons, and once you find them you can learn to replace them with true purpose and direction.

Combining my desire to help and your desire to find answers, we will walk together, as I help you through the process of reclaiming your life and learning to live with purpose, replacing your feelings of confusion, pain, anguish, and discontent with joy, happiness, clarity, and fulfillment.

At times, the journey might be difficult, but if you continue to move forward your path will become clearer. My mentor Zig Ziglar said, "Go as far as you can see, and you will see further." We will start where you are and go as far as you can. When you get there, you will be able to see a little further and continue on.

If, at any time, you feel you need professional help, please do not hesitate to reach out. If your physical or mental health is affected, please seek medical attention. Though I have learned much from life, I am not a professional counselor. Seek professional medical help if you feel suicidal or unable to shake depression or change self-defeating behaviors.

You are welcome to contact me by email if you have any questions. My email is **Janna@JannaValencia.com**.

CHAPTER 1

Know It All

I was seventeen years old and thought I knew everything. I remember standing in my grandmother's driveway and looking over the hood of my car, which was packed with all of my clothes, one foot in and one foot out, telling my mom and grandmother that I knew what I was doing, that I was going to do this my way, and to let me live my life the way I wanted to live it.

I left with nothing more than my clothes and headed to Louisiana, where my "Prince Charming" was waiting for me.

That day began a journey that would take me down some very rocky roads, not to mention some very painful experiences. By the way, as it turned out, he was definitely *not* Prince Charming.

I experienced life with him in a way I never imagined possible. We moved over and over again, finally coming back to my home town. We began to fight with each other and it became physical. I started using drugs and alcohol in an effort to make the hurt to go away and to show him I was willing to do whatever he wanted me to do so we could be together and happy. Of course, under the circumstances, none of this was possible. On the contrary, it made things much worse.

For more than twelve years I struggled, trying to make the relationship work: begging, pleading, fighting, arguing, praying, and never giving up.

I had been blessed with a wonder little girl and never wanted her to experience the pain of divorce. Because we had been having so many problems and we really did not have a secure healthy place for her to live, I had left my daughter with my grandmother.

Finally, the day came, after spending three days alone, sleeping on a mat in the back of his electronics repair shop, not having a place to shower, and not knowing how to do the repairs to get money to buy food. I was at the bottom, and I humbled myself to ask for help. I knew what was happening, but I did not want to admit it to myself or anyone else, I certainly did not want to admit I had made a mistake. I walked across our small town to the school where my mom was a teacher; it was only about three miles, although it felt like many more. The entire time, I prayed, "God, if this is not your Will he will come for me before I get there."

He did not come for me. He had left three days earlier on an excursion with the secretary he was having an affair with at the time. He was not thinking of my situation or my feelings, but I wanted to believe differently.

This was only the beginning of the end of a long battle that was full of hurt and pain, but I began to resolve that I had to do something different. I could not continue to live this way.

We went back and forth between working it out and ending the relationship. After many arguments, developing an addiction to drugs, and physical fighting that left scars on both our daughter and me, it ended badly. We had a horrible fight in front of my daughter when she was two years old that caused physical and mental pain to me and landed him in jail.

This was finally the end of that part of my life, but it was not the end of the struggle within me. I healed physically, but I was left with mental and spiritual pain, and a dangerous addiction to drugs. I was in a very delicate state, and if I did not make some dramatic changes I would end up worse than before. The separation from my husband allowed me to realize that I needed to go back to my roots and implement the values I had been raised with, but I still had to deal with the addiction that kept me from seeing clearly. This process took me away from everything I knew to be normal and familiar, but after I went through recovery I was able to see and feel again. This recovery, as you will learn in the chapters that follow, was a miracle that was given to me from God.

Even though I was gradually getting better and had begun putting my life back together, I still had not gone through the healing process, which meant walking through the necessary steps to heal, mentally and spiritually. So, in a couple of years the roller coaster started again. Over the next twenty years, I went through several relationships, all of which ended in painful loss that put me right back where I had started, alone and hurting. You would think that after the first time, I would have avoided getting into the same kind of relationship, but I couldn't avoid it because I did not understand the root of the problem.

On the surface, the relationships all looked different. They were different physically, but spiritually they were the same. Drugs and cheating, lies and gambling, followed by sexual obsessions and then extreme jealousy. The last relationship was the winner! It had many of the elements of my past relationships all rolled into one. The one thing my relationships had in common was that I longed for my partners to love me, but at the end of every relationship I would feel the same, alone and rejected.

Until I could identify the real reason I continued to attract men who were not whole themselves, I continued to experience the same results.

One day, I was sitting on the patio of my condo watching the rain fall on the lake, reflecting on my life and beginning to consider sharing my story. At that moment, I suddenly realized the reason for all the years of failure: I was looking for love and acceptance from men because of the loss I experienced when I was thirteen, which was when my parents divorced.

I was a "Daddy's Girl." I went with him everywhere. We spent countless hours together. I helped him in the field with the cows and the hay, working on the tractors and equipment, riding horses, or just taking a trip into town. We were always together.

Then one day it all stopped. I rarely saw him, and when I did it was a quick visit. We had no more quality time together. I tried living with him at one point, but he was always gone. I felt rejected and unloved. These feelings followed me for thirty years, and at the end of every relationship I entered into I had the same feelings of being rejected and unloved.

After all the years and broken relationships, I finally learned there is a process we must go through to get to the realization of what is really happening, and why. If we don't complete this process, we will relive our unsatisfying past again and again. I did.

Experience really is the best teacher, but it would have been much better if I had listened and learned from the experiences of my mother and grandmother, who tried to tell me the truth when I was only seventeen. Like many teenagers, I had to learn from my own experience.

For a long time, I lived in a cycle of depression caused by feelings of rejection and anger. This cycle resembles a figure eight lying on its side. On one side of the figure, I lived in a depressive state feeling sorry for myself, sad and hurt and looking for love. Then, when I got tired of feeling depressed, I would get angry because I felt so pitiful. I would attempt to feel better by working harder to prove myself, and by finding yet another man to prove I was worthy of love. Although I was unable to see it at the time, the cyclical motion I continually repeated was a message that there was something in me that needed to be resolved. Forget that I was in a bad relationship and had addictions, loss, or any other problems. They were the result of a deeper, underlying conflict that had to do with experiences from my childhood associated with my desire to feel love and affection.

When the cycle does not produce the desired outcome, it causes painful feelings that will manifest in different areas of your life. These feelings are internalized, and they will continue to be repeated until you realize there is an error in your behavior and you take action to change. The underlying reason for your painful feelings must be removed by accepting reality. This will allow your pain and the events that led to your pain to become the history that has created your character; instead of the circumstances that created the limiting belief that somehow you are personally deficient.

When you are living in a cyclical state, all you really want is to stop the madness and be "normal." I know this might seem impossible, but it is not. On the contrary, it is quite possible. Imagine the figure eight cycle you are revolving on as a racetrack. This track is where you place emotions that you believe will satisfy your needs. Typically, two main emotions cycle between the two ends of the figure eight; the most common are depression and anger, as discussed above. These two emotions fill some of your basic human needs and will continue cycling to fill those needs until the realization occurs and an intentional action is taken to stop the cycle.

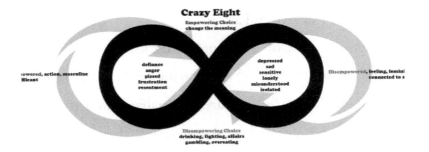

When you experience depression, it commands your entire world, including how you think, what you do, your sleeping and eating habits, and your relationships. In this state, you are likely to experience self-pity, sorrow, fear, and anxiety. You will travel on this side of the figure eight until you get tired of feeling weak, hopeless, and helpless. This is the point where the figure crosses itself and you pass into the other emotion, anger, which is the direct opposite of depression. Anger provides a false sense of strength and contentment. In this state, you feed yourself with stress and experience an intensity that drives you to be determined. You push yourself to do things that will feed your anger.

Soon you will become exhausted and pass back over and into the state of depression, and the cycle begins again. If this cycle is not broken, you will experience the same circumstances, over and over again. Your difficulties are the result of the choices you make while you are in this cycle. In order to break it, you must find a point to focus on that is higher than that in which you are currently living. This point of higher focus will be something outside of your normal life but that still exists within you. It could be creativity that is shared with others in community outreach, or it could be improving your health and relationships with your friends and family. You must find a purpose that drives your desires in an entirely different direction and begins the process that will eventually fulfill your deepest needs.

Tony Robbins and Cloe Madanes created Human Needs Psychology. Within this theory the cycles of our emotions to survive and meet our needs are explained. The Crazy Eight is one of the explanations provided in this theory and has been crucial to my understanding of the problems that I faced and has helped me break my unhealthy patterns and to fulfill my basic human needs in a healthy manner.

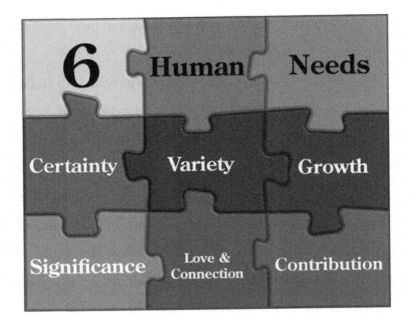

I was searching for love, but the love I found was unhealthy because it was based solely on my unfounded belief that I did not deserve to be loved. Finally, I realized that I had spent all those years looking for the love that was always there. My thoughts were in error. After my long search, I was able to feel peace, and the love that I began to experience was love without conditions.

In the following chapters we will walk through any feelings of pain, worthlessness and rejection you might be experiencing. You will learn that even in your darkest hour there is a way to survive and become victorious. You will learn how to identify your *real* problems and take the steps necessary to change the behaviors that are causing your pain. You will learn how to fill your life with a much higher purpose and gain victory over one obstacle after another, having overcome your obstacles.

It is the time to begin your "Road to Healing." Walk with me, and I will guide you through the process of turning your pain into stepping-stones that will lead to your ultimate destiny.

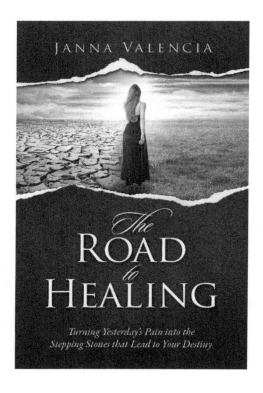

CHAPTER 2

Moving Beyond the Past

It may seem impossible to overcome the pain, so you find something that numbs you. It could be food; binging, purging, shopping, gambling, alcohol, drugs, sex, or even acts that cause you physical pain. All of these things are simply a way to remove yourself from your state of pain. The problem is twofold. First, these are temporary solutions, so when the effects of your actions are gone the pain returns. Second, these actions cause adverse effects in your life, such as relationship problems, addictions, disease, and intentional physical harm.

As I stated earlier, my drug use started out as a simple gesture to show my husband that I could be a part of his world and he could still have a good time. There were two problems with that kind of rationalization. The first was that I embraced illegal drug use, and the second was that I was throwing all of the morals and values I had been taught in the trash as I tried to fit into a situation that was against everything I truly believed. In reality, my drug use increased and quickly turned from a gesture of trying to fit in, to a necessity that began to control everything I did. The people closest to me were affected by my inconsistent, erratic behavior, and I got no closer to my husband; on the contrary, we grew further apart.

Not only did the marriage end badly, my relationship with my family suffered greatly. I didn't know what to do. As much as I wanted to stop using, the addiction controlled my every thought. I used drugs to wake up each day, to keep going throughout the day, and even to go to sleep at night. In between each use, I was only thinking about the next opportunity to use again. I neglected everything and everyone, including myself.

As with every addict who gets to the absolute bottom, I knew something had to change, but I did not know what to do. I knew if I continued to use, I would end up dead. I was lost and confused. I could have reached out to a drug counselor, family member, or a church, but I remembered my husband's mother always speaking of the love and healing power of God. In desperation, I called her to ask for help. She lived several hours from where I was living. I had to do something. I decided to take my daughter and go stay with her so she could help me. I removed myself from everything and everyone, hoping I would get better. I began to listen to her as she told me of the love of Jesus. She explained that if I trusted him, He would deliver me from the oppression and addiction that was holding me captive. I went to church with her and listened to the pastor teach about God and Jesus.

Before I ran off to live life my way, my mom always made sure we got up every Sunday morning to go to Sunday school and church service. Back then, it was one of the most dreaded days of the week. Not having options was unbearable to a rebellious teenager like me! As soon as I could figure out a way to avoid going to church, I stopped going, but the foundation had been laid. As with all well laid foundations, the storm will come, but when it passes the foundation will still be there.

During those early years, I learned about God and Jesus, but I did not know the real significance they would have in my life. At church, they spoke of the fact that Jesus died for me so I could be forgiven and have eternal life and access to all of the promises God gives us, but I did not remember any of it. When my husband's mother began to share with me and read the Bible with me, I began to hear a very different story about God and Jesus. I learned that if I asked for forgiveness and believed Jesus died to take away my sins, then I would be forgiven.

One day, I prayed, "God deliver me from this hell I'm in. Save me. I believe in you and know that you love me so much that you sent your only Son to die for me so my sins could be forgiven."

That day, He took away my sins and overlooked my shortcomings. He also delivered me from my addiction. I have never experienced another day when I wanted to use drugs.

Regardless of your situation, deliverance, peace, joy, and happiness are waiting for you. All you have to do is trust in the Father, God, and believe that He can take the burden you carry, setting you free in spite of your past.

This was not the end of the challenges I faced or the problems I would encounter; nor was I healed from my other oppressions. It was not that God didn't heal me of them, but that I didn't know I needed to be healed. I have learned that sometimes healing does not happen instantaneously, because these lessons will help you reach your ultimate destiny.

I went through life, hurt and looking for solace in other relationships, all of which were a failure. Finally, it was revealed to me that I was carrying an injury from my past, and it was time to let it go. Most often, we are not aware of what has happened, so we continue to live under these oppressions, allowing them to direct our lives.

When I finally realized that all of the years I had spent looking for peace and love in other people and drugs was really because of the hurt I carried from losing the close relationship with my father, I felt so relieved. A burden was lifted from me. At first, I felt a little ridiculous because I had spent so many years suffering over something so simple; however, I felt lighter in body and spirit, and everything around me looked brighter. All I had to do was realize the true source of my suffering and then forgive myself. Most importantly, I had to forgive my father, not for something he had done wrong, but for what I believed he had done so many years ago. You ask, "Why do you need to forgive him if he didn't do anything wrong; wasn't it just your erroneous thoughts that caused your pain?" The answer to this question is that in my mind I associated my pain with my father, whether he did anything or not. Forgiveness comes when you process your pain by releasing it through acceptance. Just as I accepted that I was a sinner and asked for forgiveness from God, I had to accept that all the years of pain from the divorce of my parents and loss of the connection with my father were just part of life in divorced families. I also needed to forgive myself for putting myself through the years of pain.

My father did not know about my feelings, nor did he have to be involved in my release of them. I had to go through the process in my own mind, and because he was linked to the pain, he would also be linked to the forgiveness.

Our minds associate people, places, and things with our experiences, which determine our thoughts, opinions, and actions. If we experience something painful, our mind will associate it with the related circumstances. In my case, my pain was associated with the absence of my father.

The next step was the process of rationalizing the association with my current knowledge. My thirteen-year-old mind did not understand that when divorce happens and jobs change, life as we know it also changes. So with this limited knowledge, I rationalized the loss of time with my father and mistakenly decided that he did not want to spend time with me anymore, and that he did not love me or want me.

When I discovered this – in the light of my new found knowledge – I realized it wasn't that he didn't love me or want to spend time with me anymore, but that he couldn't because his job had him working out of town thirty days at a time.

In Matthew 9:3-6, Jesus told the paralytic "Take courage, your sins are forgiven." He then told the scribes –who were appalled that He would say this to such a man – about the power He had to forgive by saying, which is easier, your sins are forgiven, or arise, take up your bed and go to your house." Then He instructed the man to do just that.

The same power was given to us upon His death and resurrection. As forgiveness enters as part of our life, healing begins. This example shows that forgiveness produces miraculous healing, and we should use His example to bring these same results into our own lives.

The pain you are experiencing is real, and the reasons you hurt are also real. There is, however, an area that is not real: the association you have assigned to the pain, the reason you believe you are experiencing pain.

First, you must recognize the association and the fact that it is not real. Rather, it is fiction you have created based on your knowledge of the facts. When you learn to remove the association and correct your thinking, you can remove the pain from your life and recover from it. Depending on your willingness to accept what has happened and forgive, this process can move quite rapidly, taking you almost instantly from a state of disaster to a state of contentment and happiness. Know that in spite of your past, you can live a life that is full of happiness, peace, love, joy, and prosperity.

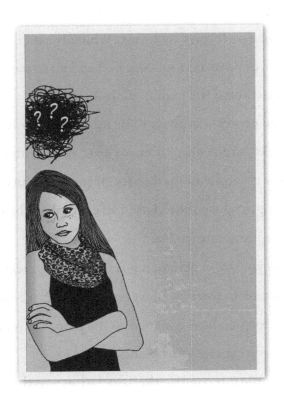

CHAPTER 3

Why God Why?

When you are going through a traumatic time in your life, the primary question you are likely to ask is "Why did this happen to me?" You just don't understand why. You only know you feel hurt, miserable, unhappy, confused, and you just want it to stop! Then, to add insult to injury, the trauma happens over and over again.

The reason your misery continues to repeat itself is because you don't see the real reasons why something happened, so you continue to relive the same experience until you come to the realization that basically yells at you, "Hey, you! Look over here! I am the reason you are living in these horrendous, vicious cycles."

There are two ways this can happened. The first is that something you experienced in the past caused your present situation. The second is that your parents or grandparents passed something to you. This is known as a "generational stronghold." Exodus 34:7 Is where this is found. Generational strongholds occur because of some sin in our parent's past that can go back as far as four generations. This is not some cult-like curse or spell that was put on you, specifically. Alcoholism is an example that is widely used. If a parent, grandparent, great-grandparent or even great, great-grandparent was an alcoholic, the sons and daughters of that person are predisposed to the stronghold of alcoholism. This stronghold will come knocking on your door, and if the door is opened you will also become an alcoholic. If you are experiencing something from your lineage, it is possible you have opened the door to a generational stronghold. This passage from the Bible documents what I am saying.

. . . .

The Lord passed in front of Moses, who proclaimed, "The Lord, the Lord, the compassionate and gracious God, slow to

*anger, abounding in love and faithfulness, maintaining love
to thousands, and forgiving wickedness, rebellion and sin.
Yet he does not leave the guilty unpunished: he punishes the
children and their children for the sin of the parents to the
third and fourth generation." Exodus, Chapter 34, 6-7 NIV*

. . . .

God tells us He is loving and faithful, but if you have done something that is sinful in His eyes and you do not ask for forgiveness and turn away from sin, it will pass to your children and your children's children up to the fourth generation. This is not an excuse to blame your parents for something that occurred in your life, but rather something that occurred in their lives is affecting you. It could also be your own actions or experiences that have created your suffering.

You can also create a generational stronghold by committing a sin and not being forgiven from it before you pass away. The stronghold you have created will then pass to the generations that follow far into the future. The important factor here is that if you have created a stronghold, you need to break it so it will not pass to future generations.

My last husband had a generational curse that was passed to him from his parents. He was constantly looking for the feeling of new love and the affection that comes with it, including the high that is experienced from sex in a new relationship. He was incapable of a healthy relationship because he was constantly living under the generational stronghold. Our relationship ended because his desire to fulfill these needs consumed him. He could not accept his situation or his responsibility for it, even though he knew he had a problem. Unfortunately, he was totally unable to commit to the process of healing.

Everyone experiences trauma. It might be from a broken relationship, addictions, loss of a loved one, physical or mental abuse, physical illness, or injury resulting in some level of disability that limits normal activity. Regardless of the type of trauma and the severity of it, two things can result. It will either be recognized, accepted, and a lesson will be learned – or it will be internalized, in which case it will cause anger, resentment, and fear to build up inside.

Hopefully, you will learn from trauma and not let it become so engrained that you become filled with negative feelings. Learning from all of your life experiences and using them to make your life better will keep you moving forward. Allowing your experiences to birth anger, resentment, and fear will cause you to repeat the same experiences over and over again. I can tell you from many years of living in such a cycle of anger and depression that this is not the option you want to take. Since you are reading this book, it's likely you've experienced the continuous cycle I'm talking about. The good news is that you do not have to live this way anymore.

The misery I experienced throughout the years – although stemming from a childhood loss – was due to the things I did to myself, not something caused by my parents or anyone else. I was looking for love from men because of the absence of my father. My addiction to drugs and alcohol was also caused by my own actions. It is important for you to take responsibility for your actions, or you will not be able to free yourself from your pain and suffering. Blaming someone else for your difficulties and refusing to accept responsibility is called *denial*, and it can only cause more hurt and pain. Now is the time to confess your sins and take responsibility for what you have done.

No matter what has happened in your life, or why, you can choose to accept it, forgive, and use the experience to create a more satisfying life. If you continue to harbor hurt inside of you and refuse to forgive, you can only become more angry and bitter, and you will attract more negative people and experiences.

Everything you do has a compound effect that works either positively or negatively. In order to understand the compound effect, I am going to use my addiction to drugs as an example.

In my first marriage, I truly thought I loved my husband. At that time, I would have done anything to keep him at my side, and I did. He used methamphetamines (meth) to get high. He was involved with the people who actually made the drug, so it was always available.

Here are the steps that led me down into drug addiction:

(Step 1) We associated with these people and they offered the drug to me.

(Step 2) I always turned it down, but at one point I decided to do what was necessary to be part of my husband's life so he would love me.

(Step 3) One day, they showed me how to take the drug without having to snort it. So...I tried it. This is how it all began.

(Step 4) One thing led to another, and I began using the drug more often and experimenting with other methods to get it into my body. In the end, I was using throughout the day to wake up, stay up, and go to sleep. All of this was to get love and affection from a man who had no idea how to love.

(Step 5) Finally, I was addicted to meth, and I had made each step into addiction of my own free will. It was not a generational stronghold caused by the actions of my parents.

If I had not stopped and asked forgiveness from God, I would have died. Even worse, I would have passed my suffering on to my daughter. It would have then passed to my precious granddaughter or one of my grandsons and to their children. What a horrible thought!

The compound effect of these small, consistent, destructive steps over time, trying to find a cure for the pain, could have caused so much more suffering in the lives of my family.

In response to the question posed at the beginning of this chapter, "Why did this happen to me?" I believe there are two reasons:

1. Situations you have experienced in your own life, and
2. Tendencies that have been passed to you from as far back as four generations.

In the process of writing this book, a friend told me a story about her son. My friend and her husband struggled with alcohol abuse and her husband's father died an alcoholic.

They were both successful in overcoming their addictions but their son struggles with alcoholism. He has been to recovery treatment twice and he also claims Jesus as his savior. What he has not done is ask God to take away the generational stronghold that was passed to him by his grandfather. My point is to show you that a generational stronghold can stay present in the family lineage even if one of the generations overcomes it. There is also the chance that one generation may not experience the stronghold because the small consistent steps that they are taking does not allow the stronghold to enter into their lives.

Reasons you do what you do:

1. To cover pain
2. To justify a feeling
3. To fit in
4. To gain acceptance
5. To gain love
6. A door was opened to a generational stronghold

You are human and have needs. When one of your needs goes unfulfilled, you will try to satisfy it with something similar. Cloe Madanes, a world renowned psychotherapist developed a program with Anthony Robbins called Strategic

Intervention. This program teaches that every person has six essential needs:

1. Certainty
2. Significance
3. Variety
4. Connection
5. Growth
6. Contribution

Although balance occurs when all of these factors are present, you are probably living in two or three of these areas more consciously than the others. These two or three needs dominate your actions. You will do what's necessary to fill them, including doing things that are hurtful and damaging to yourself and others.

For healing to occur, you must be willing to take an honest look at yourself, and then take the steps leading you to your Road to Healing.

The steps are:

1. Accept what happened.
2. Forgive yourself and others.
3. Begin to create a new you.

4. Find fulfillment and purpose in your life.

5. Give to others what you have received.

We are going to talk about each step in detail, so you can begin to overcome your past and create the stepping-stones that will lead to your true destiny.

Now that you understand there are reasons for what you are feeling, and you know there are steps you can take in order to move forward, you might still be feeling a bit uncertain. You might not believe that success is possible. I felt this way, too. It's a process that might seem daunting, at first, but we are going to process it together in small steps so you will not be overwhelmed.

You do need to know that at some point in this process memories and feelings might arise that you do not want to address or relive. I understand. Just know that if you face your pain, it can become a tool that will heal you.

Before you begin, it is necessary to understand the importance of anger and the effect it can have on your life. In the next chapter, we will talk about anger. Hopefully, you will begin to understand what it does to you and the effects it can have on your life, and the lives of those who love you.

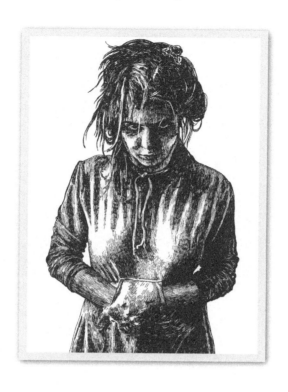

CHAPTER 4

Anger Is Making You Sick

Painful, negative experiences can cause you to become angry. Your anger can be destructive or constructive, depending on how the anger is processed. When you experience pain and hurt that is not confronted and dealt with directly, these feelings will develop into anger that can become destructive. It will dwell deep inside of you and become bitterness that will spread like cancer in your life and consume your mind with negative thoughts, mistrust, hatred, selfishness, and weakness. This weakness can give in to all of the other negativity you carry inside, manifesting in physical and mental illness.

When I experienced the hurt caused from the infidelity of my first husband, the hurt turned into anger. I took the anger and internalized it, allowing it to become bitterness. For many years, these feelings resided inside of me, along with the rejection I felt from the divorce of my parents, which, in itself, was caused by anger that had turned to bitterness. I carried that feeling into every relationship I experienced, resulting in unsatisfying and unhealthy relationships. My mental health was also affected. You see, the end result of most negative experience is anger, either with yourself or with someone else. Only you can determine whether your anger will become destructive or constructive.

You may not even know you have internalized your anger and allowed it to become bitterness, but you might recognize yourself in some of these outward signs:

1. Constant problems with others
2. Outbreaks of uncontrolled anger, rage, or fear
3. Uncontrollable actions or emotions
4. Depression
5. Recurring or unexplained illness

Your internalized anger will have an external effect on your entire life. Others can see it, but you tell yourself it is just "who you are." This is a lie you have made yourself believe. You are in control of who you are, not outside circumstances. You can allow your experiences to determine your attitude and emotions, or you can take control of them and use them in a constructive manner. When you do not deal with anger and use it constructively, you will become bitter.

How do you use anger constructively? Let's take a look at a good example of anger when it is used constructively.

It is not wrong to experience anger. This emotion is part of the human condition. Even God became angry; Jesus became angry, and because you were made in the image of God it's okay for you express anger. The problem arises when anger is allowed to control you, instead of you controlling it. 26 "In your anger do not sin": Do not let the sun go down while you are still angry, 27 and do not give the devil a foothold. 28 Anyone who has been stealing must steal no longer, but must work, doing something useful with their own hands, that they may have something to share with those in need. 29 Do not let any unwholesome talk come out of your mouths, but only what is helpful for building others up according to their needs, that it may benefit those who listen. 30 And do not grieve the Holy Spirit of God, with whom you were sealed for the day of redemption. 31 Get rid of all bitterness, rage and anger, brawling and slander, along with every form of malice." Ephesians 4: 26-31 God and Jesus used anger to teach and correct, but they had intention to harm. On the contrary, they used strong actions to show where a wrong had occurred, and then they explained why it was wrong. For example, one time Jesus went into the temple at Passover and found the people trading and money changing. The temple was a holy place for God, not a place to conduct business. It angered Jesus, and He began throwing the tables being used for the trading out of the temple. He exclaimed that the temple was His Father's house and should not be defiled by turning it into a house of trade. (John 2:13-23)

26 "In your anger do not sin": Do not let the sun go down while you are still angry...31 Get rid of all bitterness, rage and anger, brawling and slander, along with every form of malice." Ephesians 4:26 & 31

The actions of Jesus harmed no one, but He got the attention of the people performing the trading so He could teach them it was wrong, and why. He did not hold a grudge

against these people, but forgave them and continued to love them. You need to do the same.

Right now, you might be thinking, "You really don't understand what I went through, or you would not be telling me to give up holding a grudge!" Believe me, I understand. I felt the same way. In my case, there were countless other women, lie after lie, constant deceit, loss of material and immaterial possessions. I completely understand! I felt alone and believed there was no one I could turn to. I did not understand why it was happening or what I did to deserve it. I couldn't understand why men treated me so badly and did terrible things to me. All I knew was I hurt, and although I didn't want everyone to know it, I spread my bitterness around in the form of mistrust of others and I made false statements. I had fits of anger arising from my misguided attempts to protect myself and prove I was not weak and could control my own life. I didn't discriminate against anything or anyone who crossed my path. The entire time, I justified my actions and blamed *others* for what I had become.

The truth is that no one made me into a person who was angry and bitter. I had been hurt and didn't want to deal with it, so I "stuffed it" as far down inside of me as I could. This way I did not have to feel the pain. When I was in the state of anger, I felt strong, in control, and determined. Because of the false sense of security it gave me, I held onto it tightly. As a result, I walked around with bitterness inside of me for many years, always attracting more of it because I refused to deal with it and let it go.

On the flip side of anger, I entered into periods of depression. In one of my failed relationships, my partner was so obsessed with sex and pornography that I tried to take his mind off of it by becoming like the women he was obsessed with. I could not really *be* one of those women; it was completely against my nature to act that way, and it caused me to feel ugly, dirty, and rejected. I withdrew, and in my depression I was so miserable I gained almost 100 pounds. At a tremendous 225 pounds, I felt horrible inside and looked horrible on the outside. I was mentally ill and physically sick all of the time. Then, to top it all off, I would eat to comfort myself and gain more weight.

Finally, it was enough! I ended the relationship and, once again, started working to put my life back together. I began walking to a local park with my daughter, where we played tennis. I started going to church and getting involved with activities there. I also began to watch what I ate. I lost 75 of the nearly 100 pounds over a period of time and felt better about myself. There was just one thing I didn't do: let go of my anger and bitterness. I just put it down inside me and let it continue to build. Not long after that I married again, thinking it was going to be a lasting relationship.

He was a wonderful person with a huge heart but he was hurt and angry, too. Of course, over time, the vicious cycle repeated itself, and I stuffed more loss, hurt, rejection, pain, anger, and bitterness inside. Where would it all end? When would I finally learn? Change was coming, but my dilemma was not resolved until ten years later, when I finally realized that to achieve my ultimate destiny I had to let go of all the unhealthy habits I was holding onto.

Drugs, alcohol, sex, arguing, fighting, jealousy, deceit, and lies – none of it was who I really wanted to be. But I was holding on to all of it, and it was oozing out of me, making me and others think I was someone who, in reality, I was not. My anger and destructive actions were attracting more of the same, until I finally did something different. Instead of chasing a man to fill my inner void, I stopped living in protective mode and running through cycles of feeling depressed and angry. I began looking for the real reasons for my negative behaviors. This started with one small step in the right direction. I was ready for change.

One day, as I was thumbing through my Facebook page, I saw a post from Tom Ziglar. It was a short video that explained how he was continuing the legacy of his father by teaching others to deliver his father's message. His father was Zig Ziglar. I grew up listening to Zig Ziglar's message because my mom played his tapes when we rode in her car. Something told me I should pursue this, so I submitted the form for them to call me. Soon they called to give me all of the details. I knew I had to pursue this course of study. Something inside of me leapt with joy and determination when I talked or thought about it. I went to the training and was gone for a week. When I came home, I was already beginning to feel a change. I saw things differently, and people saw me differently.

A few months later, my husband left. Once again, I was confronted with the same rejection and feelings of being unloved. This time, although difficult, I saw it differently. I began to reflect on all the years of constant battles in my relationships and the similarities of all of them. I did not want this time to be the same as all the others.

Once more, I turned to the One who is always faithful and just to forgive and to love without condition. I looked to a higher power to give me hope, Jesus. This time, I truly accepted all that He had to give me, and I released all that I was holding onto. I let Him take all of it from me. I cannot explain the feeling I had when I let Him take complete control of my life and reveal to me each of the instances where there had been sin, hurt, and pain. As each one was revealed, He removed it from within me. I felt the weight being lifted and light beginning to shine within me. This did not happen all in one day, but over the course of a few months. I recalled each experience, one at a time, dealing with the pain and allowing it to be accepted as part of my past. I must tell you, this was not the only time I had asked Jesus to take my suffering from me, and it was not the first time He took it. But it was the first time I let go.

If you let go of your suffering, He will take it from you, and you will feel what I am explaining to you now.

. . . .

Jesus said, "Come to me all ye who are weary and burdened, and I will give you rest. Take my yoke upon you and learn from me, for I am gentle and humble in heart, and you will find rest for your souls. For my yoke is easy and my burden is light." Matthew 11: 28-30 NIV

. . . .

I needed rest for my soul. What about you? You do not have to keep bitterness inside of you anymore. Give it to Him, so you can heal and find peace.

When I began to discover my own healing, I started reading many articles and studies about how anger causes physical and mental illness. In thinking back on my experiences, in addition to myself I could identify more than one person who had made themselves physical and mentally sick because of anger and bitterness. At the time, I did not understand. I just knew something was not right. It's amazing how many of us decide to blame someone or something else for our circumstances, when, in reality, we have allowed the circumstances of our past to determine our future.

Begin today. If you are willing to let go of past hurts you will find peace. First, you will have to go through a process to retrain your mind and allow your heart to heal. It starts with acknowledging and accepting that something destructive happened to you, either because of a bad choice that you made or something that you had no control over it at the time.

CHAPTER 5

Step 1: Acceptance

E veryone has experienced something in their life that was painful and made them angry. Some dealt with it well by accepting what happened. They used it as a tool to better themselves physically, mentally, and spiritually.

If you have let your pain and anger become bitterness, it is likely you will live with it until you can't take it any longer. When you get to this point, you will feel like there is no other place to turn and nothing you can do. Consider the helplessness we all felt the dreadful morning of September 11, 2001, the day America stood still. Everyone was in a state of shock. No one could believe what had just happened, nor could they understand why. That day is still so vivid in my mind and heart. My soul still feels the pain of all the people who lost family members and loved ones. Afterwards, the majority of

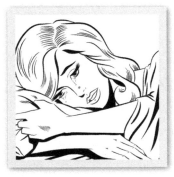 Americans, including me, walked around in a state of numbness, disbelief, helplessness, and even fear. Those who lost loved ones felt all of this, in addition to the pain of loss. I can remember the feeling of helplessness that I experienced that day because our country was now at risk, there was so many people who needed help but we could not get to them fast enough and because of the families who were directly affected by this tragedy. Although I did not directly lose anyone, I felt the pain for those who did.

When you feel as if you have no reason to keep living, and you are at the lowest of lows and gripped by fear and depression, you can make changes in your life. When you have exhausted every personal capability you have and are ready to accept the help that is being offered, you will do whatever is necessary to move forward in a new, more positive direction.

You might not know you are at this point, but something will trigger you and jolt you out of your current state of mind and into a different state of being or feeling. This sudden jolt will not feel "normal." It will be outside of your usual cycle of progression from anger to depression.

In this changed state, you will be ready to let go of your past suffering. You will begin to forgive yourself and take the first step toward your healing and true purpose.

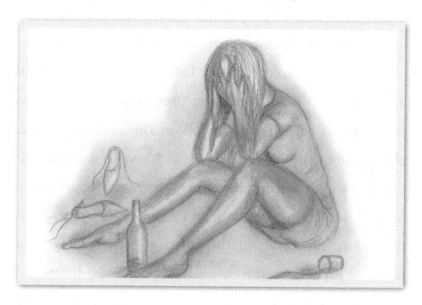

ADDICTION

If you are or have been addicted to drugs, alcohol, sex, gambling, or anything else that controls your thoughts and actions, and you are ready to accept that you are helpless and unable to control your life, I urge you to reach out to someone who can hold you accountable to your decision to accept that you cannot control your physical and mental desire to use or partake in your particular addiction.

Speak these words out loud to yourself or another person:

"I am helpless and unable to control _____ (fill in the blank with your addiction), and I am willing to accept that I am helpless. I want and need help to overcome my addiction, and I will commit to getting better today." Do this every day until you no longer have the desire to feed your addiction.

In addition to accepting your inability to do it alone, you must separate yourself from any environment that encourages you to participate in your addiction. This includes people, places, and situations. The people you normally use with will not help you stop using; the places you visited to participate in your addiction will continue to encourage your addiction. Don't go there! Anything that might encourage you to use or participate in your addiction is now off-limits. An example would be to refrain from using the Internet if you are addicted to sex or gambling, because it's an easy access point for indulging in these activities.

Addiction is a habit. All humans have habits. The difference is that habits can be productive or destructive. Any habit that alters the state of your mind into numbness, exaggerated thinking or feeling, changes your thought process, or is physically dangerous for you and your health are not good habits.

In order to change an addiction or negative habit, you must replace it with a new habit. The new habit should be very different from your former habit. It should offer healthy options. To begin to replace these habits, you will need a support group. This does not have to be a professional group, but your chances of success will be much higher if you choose to incorporate professional support into your recovery. Your addiction is the result of your need to fill one of the six basic human needs because one or more of your needs is not being met. When you satisfy your needs with something positive, your desire to partake in addiction will diminish.

I also encourage you to get involved with a church that offers help for addicts. It is necessary to connect with a higher power to help you release your negative feelings.

When I was going through the process of recovery, I submerged myself in the love and word of God. As a result, I was delivered from my addiction. With the added strength and support of your higher power, you can recover and become whole again. Jesus has and continues to deliver many people from the oppression that has held them captive. He has forgiven many from the sins they committed while they were blinded by oppression. You are no different. If you will reach out to Him and ask Him to forgive you, He will. There is nothing more powerful than knowing you can let go of your addictions and the experiences that caused them.

> *You will again have compassion on us; you will tread our sins underfoot and hurl all our iniquities into the depths of the sea. Micah 7:19 NIV*

You no longer need to live in bondage to your addictions. You have the healing power of Jesus at your disposal. The only thing you need to do is ask for His help and stand firm as you call on His power, resisting oppression and temptation when it knocks on your door.

Be aware that even with the glory of healing and deliverance, there is another side that does not want you to be free. Your body and mind will crave whatever you are addicted to. This oppression will try to regain control of you, and if you allow it all the progress you've made will be lost, and you will have to start over.

The good news is that all you need to do is resist the

temptation to indulge in your addiction, and it will hold less and less power over you. Eventually, it will become easy to resist, and you will be stronger and more liberated.

Submit yourselves therefore to God. Resist the devil,
and he will flee from you. James 4:7 KJV

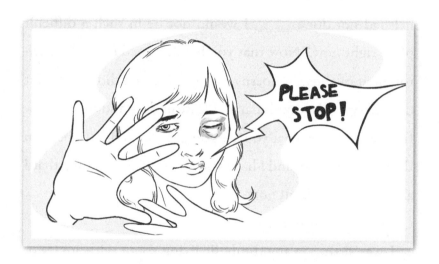

ABUSE

If you are in an abusive situation, find an opportunity to separate yourself from the person who is abusing you and go directly to a shelter or church that helps abuse victims. Do not leave notes or communicate with the abuser for any reason. If you have borne children with this person, take the children with you. Once you are in a safe place, the counselor or pastor will help you to take the next steps to remove yourself permanently from the abuser.

At this point, you must begin the process of acceptance. The abuse happened and there is nothing that you can do to change this fact. Accept it and let it be okay. Most importantly, avoid making statements like, "If I had done _____, or if I had not done _____, I would not be in such a difficult place right now." Now that you have escaped from the environment of abuse, it doesn't matter what you did, or did not do. Perhaps this sounds harsh. Please understand that I know from experience what you are going through. I have been in the same position, and I have said and done everything that I am telling you about now.

This was my experience:

I was sitting in my dimly lit living room with my two-year-old daughter, who was sleeping on the loveseat across the room. I was soaring from the high of methamphetamine.

Suddenly, there was a startling noise of someone kicking the door, and before I realized what was happening another swift kick brought the front door of the house crashing open. My estranged husband, the father of my daughter, came rushing into the living room. He grabbed me by the hair and began hitting me, pulling me through the house by my hair and screaming horrible profanities. My little girl was terrified. I had to do something to stop him. I began to fight back in an attempt to free myself and get my daughter away from the horror of the experience.

At that moment, my younger sister "just happened" to come by the house, and she called my grandparents, who lived only one mile away. This was really an intervention of God. My husband ran out of the house, which gave me a reprieve from the blows.

I thought he was leaving, but he had gone to his truck and come back with a gun! I really did not know if he would shoot me, but I was reeling in pain and confusion. My sister told him that she had called the police and they were on their way. It was my good fortune that he left.

This incident was the beginning of the end of that particular abusive relationship. It was not easy, but it was necessary. I was living in a small town and there was nowhere to go to get away from him. Strung out, scared, and afraid, I went to the home of my grandparents because they were close friends with the Sheriff, who sent regular patrol around the house until they could find him and put him in jail.

I was at the bottom, as low as anyone could go. Knowing

that I needed to do something, and not knowing what, I began to listen to the voice inside me that told me to leave. I didn't know if it right or not. All that I knew was that my lifestyle was going to kill me if something didn't change. So, as I mentioned earlier, I left and went to live with my mother-in-law. She was a wonderful woman who loved God, and I believed she would help me to overcome my difficulties. She did help me overcome my addictions, and she made sure I was safe from my husband, although, by that time, he had decided to pursue one of the women he'd had an affair with and he really had no more interest in me. This was a real miracle, even though I did not see it at the time.

I had no idea how I was going to overcome the pain I felt from my broken relationship, but I began to focus on recovery. I received Christ as my personal savior, and He delivered me from my addiction to methamphetamines. From that day, I have never had an uncontrollable desire to use again. This is not to say that I was not presented with the opportunity or did not think about it, but I was no longer weak. I was able to turn away and resist it, and I never put myself in an abusive situation again.

During the time we were together, my husband would say things that were not true, but I believed them. These things were degrading and they made me feel bad about myself. This is quite common in abusive relationships. The abuser will degrade you until you have no self-worth and you are totally dependent on him (or her). This is how you are controlled and kept in the abusive relationship.

From a spiritual view, addiction and abuse are forms of oppression that are used by the forces of darkness, also called Lucifer, the devil or Satan, to control us and keep us from experiencing all of what Jesus has to offer.

*Be alert and of sober mind. Your enemy the
devil prowls around like a roaring lion looking
for someone to devour. 1 Peter 5:8 NIV*

These oppressions will dominate your life and destroy you if you do not take action. Begin your recovery today and walk in freedom from your past. All is not lost; on the contrary, this can be the beginning of a beautiful journey that will bring you to the state of mind you have desired for so long. It may seem like there is no way out, but I am living proof there is always a way to change. If I can do it, you can, too. You are not alone in this journey, and if you will allow it, Jesus will walk beside you, talk with you, and even carry you when you cannot find the strength to do it yourself.

So do not fear, for I am with you; do not be dismayed, for I am your God. I will strengthen you and help you; I will uphold you with my righteous right hand. Isaiah 41:10 NIV

You are worthy, you are blessed, you are beautiful, you are joyful, you are intelligent, you are capable, you are strong, and most of all, you are loved. Let all of the past be the past. Begin to embrace a new and brighter future that is full of everything you desire in your heart. Accept the things that have happened and know they are in the past. Nothing can prevent you from moving forwards on your personal Road to Healing and reaching your ultimate destiny.

LOSS

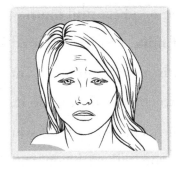

If you have ever experienced loss due to divorce, death, or destruction, you have experienced significant pain, anger, and grieving.

My young adulthood was spent living in grief from the loss

of my father after my parent's divorce when I was thirteen. I carried this grief throughout my adult life, searching for relief in other men but never finding it. I also lost my sister in a terrible auto accident. Her two young children and her husband also died in the accident. There are really no words to explain such a loss. Losing a loved one through tragedy is especially difficult because there is no warning. It leaves you with a helpless feeling because there is no chance for closure. Loss of a loved one from illness or disease is also difficult, but the difference is that usually there is time for closure. This is not to say it's any easier, just that there is time to express your love and say goodbye.

Loss is a part of life and everyone experiences it to some degree. Processing loss and turning it into a positive force will give you a deeper level of understanding and appreciation of life and other people. If you allow loss to consume you, death and regret will affect you in negative ways. Accept your loss and allow it to enrich your life with beautiful memories. Let it be an experience that teaches you that your life is part of a higher plan, one you cannot know or understand. God's plan for us is always perfect.

*For My thoughts are not your thoughts, nor are your
ways My ways, declares the Lord. For as the heavens are
higher than the earth, so are My ways higher than your
ways and My thoughts than your thoughts. For as the
rain and the snow come down from heaven, and do not
return there without watering the earth and making it
bear and sprout, and furnishing seed to the sower and
bread to the eater; so will My word be which goes forth
from My mouth; It will not return to Me empty, without
accomplishing what I desire, and without succeeding in
the matter for which I sent it. Isaiah 55:8-11 NIV*

Perhaps you have never been told about Jesus and the significance of His life. Jesus is the Son of God, our maker and the maker of the universe and all that is in it. God made us in His image, and He loves us as He loves His own child, Jesus. He originally made man and then woman to be his partner, but they were deceived by the Devil and condemned to life separate from God. So God sent His son Jesus to earth to live as a man, grow as a man, and experience earthly life. The difference is that Jesus was without sin. He died on a cross and shed His blood for us to cover our sins so we could again be in communion with God, who is our Father.

* *

For God so loved the world that he gave His only
begotten Son, that whosoever believeth in Him
should have everlasting life. John 3:16 KJV

* *

You can know the joy and love of Jesus Christ and have the comfort of knowing that He is always with you. All you must do is accept Him as your Savior by simply acknowledging that you believe He is the Son of God and that He died for you on the cross so you could be saved. Ask Him to forgive you for your sins and come into your heart and wash you clean. He *will* be faithful to come and remove the pain of your abuse or the misery of your addiction and give you eternal life. He does not discriminate, and it doesn't matter what happened to you or what you have done. He loves you and wants you to accept Him into your life, so He can comfort and love you with His unconditional love.

RELATIONSHIPS

We experience several types of relationships, including:

1. Familial (family)
2. Platonic (friends)
3. Romantic (love)
4. Professional (business)

Relationships can bring you much joy and meet many of your needs. They can also cause you much pain. Most of us try to meet our needs in whatever way we can. Depending on how we seek to fulfill them, sometimes we expose ourselves to problems and situations that can haunt us for years.

When loss or other major disturbance occurs in a family, a chain reaction can occur, leading to a lifetime of difficulties if the emotions involved are not uncovered and released. As described earlier, this was my experience.

Platonic relationships are basically friendships that can include different levels of intimacy. In most platonic relationships, we begin as acquaintances and grow into being friends as trust develops. As time passes, your friend can become a trusted confidant and will feel like part of the family. When this trust is betrayed, you can become fearful and withdraw from making new friends.

In my first marriage, one of my closest friends from high school slept with my husband. This caused me to withdraw from making new friends with women, because I did not want to experience anything like that again. For many years I could not trust other women, especially around the men in my life. This experience caused me to feel the same rejection I felt when I lost my father.

I also experienced levels of similar betrayal in my professional relationships and, of course, everyone knows about the romantic relationships.

When I was a small child, I spent many hours at my grandparent's house because my parents were working. My grandparents loved to entertain and had many friends, who would come to the house each week to play cards. My siblings and I wanted to be part of the party, too, but my grandparents would always tell us "children should be seen and not heard." This was one way they taught us to respect our elders. There was nothing wrong with what they did, but this repeated statement caused me to associate being good with not speaking, and I had a difficult time approaching a person older than myself until I was in my thirties. I did not understand why, and it caused frustration because I was unable to excel in some areas of my work because my brain had been programmed with this particular thought pattern.

You see, it does not matter what kind of relationship you have, it can still cause pain that results in anger, which can cause bitterness and ultimately illness. Until you release your anger, hopefully with the help of God, you will continue to live within the "crazy eight" (described in an earlier chapter) in a negative attempt to fulfill your needs. The cycle will fill some of your needs for certainty, significance, love/connection, and variety, but it will never fill all of them, leaving you searching and feeling frustrated and angry, including anger at yourself for your perceived "failure."

As you revolve in the cycle, you might feel hopeless, but there is always hope. The answer lies in acknowledging and accepting the painful events in your past.

The next step is forgiveness. This might be difficult, and you might struggle with it. But if you are able to forgive those who have hurt you, the hardest part will be over. The world will begin to look different, opening avenues of possibilities that you might not have known about. Join me now and get past the hardest part. Break through into new experiences and your bright new future.

Chapter 6

Step 2: Forgiveness

You have made it to the most difficult step you will take in this process. There are some painful experiences you have held onto and still have running rampant through your heart. Your mind will try to control your thinking. It will tell you the person who has abused you does not deserve to be forgiven, and that all of the things that happened are too much to forgive. You harbor an attitude of unforgiving and use it as a safety net, but it is time to let it go.

Healing can only begin when you empty your heart of the

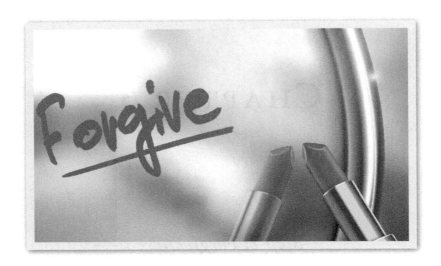

darkness and pain you keep inside. This means you must look at yourself in the mirror and tell yourself: "I deserve better. I am beautiful, blessed, intelligent, and loved. Most of all, I am the child of a King." You are "royalty," so you need to accept it and let this knowledge replace the painful, destructive thoughts you are holding on to.

. . . .

For you are all children of God, by faith in Jesus Christ. Galatians 3:26 NIV

. . . .

Forgiveness comes when you have truly accepted that everything in your life is merely a series of events, positive and negative, and that you can use your experiences to become a stronger person. Let your experience become part of your good character. I say "good" character because what you have experienced can reflect in both good and bad ways. These experiences will mold your character, but you do not have to let them mold you negatively. If something has affected you negatively, you can overcome it and reverse the "curse," if you will. Whatever happened is in the past. You cannot change it, but you can use it to give you insight and help you make future decisions.

Many years after the lies and cheating I endured with my first husband's affairs, I held every other man up to this original example. I was unable trust any of them. It isn't that I didn't want to trust them; it's just that I couldn't trust them. I had so many bad memories running on automatic replay in my mind, and when something triggered one of these memories I would react accordingly. This caused many problems and a lot of confusion in my subsequent relationships. Although I was a caring, trusting person behind the façade, all the "cargo" I was carrying around made me cold and untrusting.

Throughout the years, I met many people who were afraid of me. I always wondered why. One time, someone had the courage to tell me what she thought when I asked this question. She told me it was because of the way I carried myself. She explained that I seemed rigid and strict, and because I held positions of leadership in my career, people would not get close to me for fear they would say or do something that would cause conflict or they would lose their job. The real reason people saw me this way is because I was walking around with this fake outward appearance to protect myself from being hurt again.

I carried this around with me for many years, until I finally I came to the realization that even though I was saved, and Jesus had healed me the day I received Him into my heart, I had not let Him take everything from me. Have you ever cried out to God saying, "Oh God, please take this from me! I don't want it anymore! It hurts too much! I can't take it anymore!" I cried out to Him in this way many times, and every time He took my suffering from me.

But if He had taken away my pain, why did I still carry it around and continue to experience it? The answer is simple. When I cried out, He was faithful to come and take it away to make my burden lighter, but once I felt better I held on to my pain instead of leaving it at the feet of Jesus.

. . . .

"Come to me, all you who are weary and burdened, and I will give you rest. Matthew 11:28 NIV

. . . .

His promise to all of us is that He will take our burdens and give us His peace. Imagine how He had to forgive those who crucified him. The people, who He loved dearly, chose to release a known murderer back into their midst, yet they hung Jesus on a cross. (You can read this story in Matthew, Chapter 27.)

Even though you say and do things that hurt Him, He is faithful to forgive you of it all. If Jesus could do it for you, then you should be able to do it for yourself and those who have wronged you.

Forgiveness releases the anger that has turned to bitterness inside you. It will relieve you of the burden you carry. This burden is heavy and can make you physically and mentally ill. You must come to understand the reality that holding on to pain and hurt will not make anything better. It will not protect you from future hurt; on the contrary, it will prevent you from experiencing what you need and desire. It is not possible to find what you long for in the midst of chaos, malice, dissention, and deceit, even though you are longing for the direct opposite: peace, love, tranquility, and truth.

To begin forgiving yourself and others, I suggest you start with the first person who comes to your mind. As you begin to tick off the hurtful incidents and empty your heart and mind of these experiences, others will begin to surface. As you remember them, forgive the other person, but also forgive yourself. I want to stress this point, because if you continue to beat yourself up over problems from your past and are unable to forgive yourself, you will not be able to truly forgive anyone else. Think about it. You can say, "I forgive you," but what does it really mean if you still feel lousy because of the abuse and you are continually saying to yourself that you were stupid for_____ (fill in the blank). Accusation is a sign of an inability to forgive. You must let it go. It happened and it cannot be changed. You have held onto it not knowing you were really causing yourself more pain. Jesus forgave you for harboring past events and suffering, and he forgave the other people who were involved for the part they played. If He can do it for you, then you can do it for yourself.

I began by forgiving my first husband for his infidelity and physical abuse, because he was the first person who came up. Next, I forgave my most recent husband for his infidelity and lies. Then my other relationships began to come up, and one by one I forgave them. When the most obvious were dealt with, much to my surprise, I began to remember many other events from my past that were so deeply buried I had not remembered them. I forgave each one.

Finally, I began to relive my relationship with my father and the pain I felt from the times when I wanted to see him and he wasn't there. It haunted me for days. I didn't understand why, but then it dawned on me. I was still suffering from losing the closeness we once had. This was something deep inside of me. It was nothing my father had done; it was not his fault. But the hurt from his leaving had become anger and then bitterness. I had to get it out of me. I had to forgive him for leaving, even though he never knew about the pain I experienced, it was never his intention for me to be hurt.

Some of you might have had similar experiences that were even more traumatic. Perhaps something happened in your youth that really hurt you, and you have held it inside for many years. No one but you, the other person involved, and God know about it. What happened to you seems unpardonable. Listen to me now! There is nothing more important than to process your pain and begin to forgive. Don't close your mind. The inability to forgive is the one thing that holds you captive. It will continue to control your life with one bad experience after another, one hit after another, one more drink, one more relationship, and one more new start. It's time to recover, to be healed, to regain your life and be happy, healthy, prosperous, and truly loved. Stay with me, and we will walk through this together. It will not be easy, but you can, and will, get through it.

. . . .

It's time to recover, to be healed, to regain your life and be happy, healthy, prosperous, and truly loved.

. . . .

The following is a story told by a world-renowned minister, Joyce Meyer. I want you to know this story because she is a perfect example of someone who endured the unbearable and is now living her ultimate destiny and true purpose.

Joyce Meyers, a well know evangelist tells her story about her life of abuse by her father. This is her story. Her father sexually, mentally, emotionally, and verbally abused her as far back as she can remember, until she left home at the age of eighteen. He did many terrible things...some of which are too distasteful for her to talk about publicly. But she wants to share her testimony because so many people have been hurt, and they need to realize that someone has made it through the same struggles so they can have hope.

More than anything, she wants you to know and really understand that anyone who has been abused can fully recover if they will give their life completely to Jesus.

Abuse is defined as "to be misused, used improperly, or to be wasted; to use in such a way as to cause harm or damage; to be treated cruelly." Any time we are misused or used for a purpose other than what God intended, it's damaging. Many people can relate to this. For some of you reading this, Joyce is just telling your story. You know what it's like to live with a terrible, shameful secret that is eating you alive.

Her father was a mean, controlling, and manipulative person for most of his life. He was unpredictable and unstable. As a result, the atmosphere of their home was supercharged with fear, because they never knew if what they did would make him mad or not.

They always did what he wanted to do, when he wanted to do it. They watched what he wanted to watch on TV, went to bed when he went to bed, got up when he got up, and ate the meals he wanted them to eat...everything in their home was determined by his moods and what he wanted.

The sexual abuse started when she was very young, and when he decided she was mature enough he took things even further. From that point until she was eighteen, he raped her at least once a week. Her father, who she was supposed to be able to trust and who was supposed to keep her safe, was the person she came to fear the most.

She was profoundly ashamed because of this. She was ashamed of herself, of her father and what he did. She was also constantly afraid. There was no place that ever felt safe while she growing up. She explains that believe that we cannot even begin to imagine what kind of damage this does to a child.

She pretended to have a normal life, but she felt lonely all the time and different from everyone else. She never felt like she fit in. She was not allowed to participate in after-school activities, go to sports events or parties, or date boys. Many times, she had to make up stories about why she couldn't do anything with her classmates. She lived with pretense and lies for a long time.

What she learned about love was actually perversion. Her father told her what he did to her was special and because he loved her. He said everything he did was good, but it had to be their secret because no one else would understand and it would cause problems in the family. It became Joyce's burden not to let her pain cause problems in her family. However, as long as she kept the secret, she couldn't get free from the pain of it.

You may be wondering where God was in all of this. He was there. He didn't get her out of the situation when she was a child, but He did give her the strength to get through it. Her father abused her and did not love and protect her the way he should have, and at times she felt as no one would ever help her and it would never end.

But God always had a plan for her life and He has redeemed her. He has taken what Satan meant for harm and turned it into something good (see Romans 8:28). He has taken away her shame and given her a double reward and recompense (see Isaiah 61:7).

It may seem impossible, but God's truth set her free from a life of pretense and lies. His truth has restored her soul and made her living proof that nothing is too hard for God. No matter what you have been through or how bad you hurt, there is hope!

"That's why I'm telling my story. You need to know how good God is and that your struggle is worth it. If you will give your life to Christ and really trust God, you can be completely healed and restored so you can live the life Jesus died for you to have. Don't give up!" Joyce Meyers

On the flip side of this horrible reality is that the pain you experienced was from your own perception, unlike the story above in which the abuser knew it was wrong but did nothing to stop. The other people involved might not have been aware that you were damaged. However, you carry this around with you and it becomes part of you. When you realize the person, or persons, involved in the experience did not hurt you intentionally, and that holding on to your pain has directed your life in unproductive and negative ways, you might feel really dumb. But, eventually, you will feel a lot of relief from knowing the harm was never intentional. Then, you will be able to forgive.

After I had dealt with my experience of abuse, and I had been relieved from all the years of pain and hurt, I began to see more clearly. I believed the process was finished and that I had forgiven everyone who had played a part in the drama (including myself), but I was quite wrong. I began to remember things that happened that I had not remembered in many years. These were things that were hurtful, such as statements people had made that were not true, events that happened that I did not want to happen but they did anyway, and things I did that later I regretted but couldn't take back. All of these situations had a bearing on my inability to forgive others and myself.

When long forgotten experiences begin to present themselves and, once again, you are reliving them, don't stop moving forward. Forgive yourself and the others involved, and continue moving towards your ultimate destiny. Don't get stuck on any event or person and try to figure out why. It doesn't matter. This was something that happened and it cannot be changed. Constantly remind yourself that to forgive is to live in truth and honesty, and that as you continue to remove these things from your heart you will begin to heal and every step will bring you closer to becoming whole again.

When long forgotten experiences begin to present themselves and, once again, you are reliving them, don't stop moving forward. Forgive yourself and the others involved, and continue moving towards your ultimate destiny.

One last thing I want to remind you of is that you are not alone in any of this process. Whether you have decided to let Jesus into your heart to be your Savior, or not, He is there. He is always watching, and if ever you feel alone just ask Him to come into your heart. You will feel His love and warmth instantly.

CHAPTER 7

Step 3: Creating A New You

You have been through so much and worked so dili-gently to take back control of your life. You are begin-ning to feel good and see light where before there was only darkness. It is time to start building your new life. This journey will not happen overnight, but if you are willing to begin

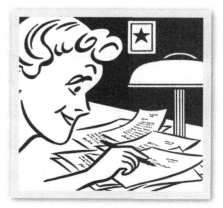

planning and creating a new life for yourself it will manifest. Many people who come out of addictions, abusive situations, and loss often stop at this point, because they feel relieved, to some degree. However, this is not the time to stop; on the contrary, it's time to start. You have come a long way and have made a lot of progress, but now you need to put new purpose into your life and fill it with all of the things you desire.

Start by having a "dreaming session." Everyone dreams of what they want to achieve for themselves and their families. You, too, can have everything you want. Start by taking a sheet of paper and writing down everything you can think of that you want to create. Don't limit yourself. Don't ask someone else to help you. Just dream and write it down. Let me help you get started.*

What would you like to do with your life? Maybe you would like to create a new career or get a college degree. Perhaps you would like to open a business of your own.

What about material possessions? Do you want a home of your own, a bigger house or a new car? Perhaps you would like to take a vacation and travel around the world.

---

* A Dream Sheet is included in the appendix to write down all of your dreams.

What about your relationships? If you are not already married, would you like to be? If so, what does your new spouse look like, and what characteristics do they possess? For example, are they funny, compassionate, handsome, romantic, or wealthy? What's important to you in a mate?

Let's talk about your new friendships and the people who surround you. It's very important that you begin to form new relationships with like-minded people. These people should encourage your new, healthier lifestyle and help you continue moving forward. They should be willing to hold you accountable for staying on the right track. It's easy to let yourself return to past negative habits such as drug addition. It's important to keep reminding yourself why you decided to make changes in your life. The people you have contact with every day should model the new life you are building. They should support you in your endeavors. I am not saying they should agree with everything you say or do, but they should encourage you to keep growing stronger, healthier, and wiser in making decisions. While you are in the process of healing, your mind, body, and soul are like a sponge soaking in all of the outside support or opposition you come into contact with. In order to continue to heal, you must take in as much positive support as you can. It's not possible to live without opposition, but it is possible to overcome and not succumb to negativity.

Your dreams are the goals you have decided to work towards. Now that you have written them down, it's time to categorize them and determine which goals you want focus on. First, determine what area of your life the dream is related to.

There are seven areas in which to categorize your dreams[†]:

1. Family
2. Personal
3. Mental
4. Spiritual
5. Professional
6. Health
7. Financial

Every dream you have is likely to be in one of these categories. If your dream is to find a spouse or have children, this would be in the family category. If you want to start a business, this would be in the professional category. If you are an addict who is recovering, perhaps one of your dreams

---

[†] Categorize your dreams on the worksheet titled "Categorize My Dreams" sheet found in the appendix.

is to overcome needing a drink or a fix every day. This would in the mental category.

Now that your dreams are categorized, we are going to determine if they are dreams you really want to achieve or if they are what we call "pipe dreams." These are goals that really don't benefit you or anyone else who might be involved. With this in mind, ask yourself this question related to each dream:

"Is it good, right, and just for everyone involved?"

If the answer is "Yes," then this particular goal can pass to the next phase. If the answer is "No," you will not be able to move this dream to the next phase. This does not mean that at some point in the future you cannot move it to the next phase, but it's not a good idea at the beginning. Remember, you are still healing and forming a life that is wholesome, healthy, and good. If something doesn't fit into your new life, then you should get rid of it and replace it with something that is.

MY WHY[‡]

The next phase in qualification of your goals is to determine

‡ A worksheet titled MY WHY is included for you to write all of the passionate reasons you want to achieve your goals in the appendix

how excited or passionate you feel about each particular one. When you think about this dream how does it make you feel? How much time can you spend thinking about it? Does it wake you up at night? Do you wake up thinking about it?

If you are not passionate about your dream or goal, you will not be dedicated to completing it when obstacles arise. Alternatively, if you are consumed by the idea of achieving the dream, and you can see yourself being it, doing it, or having it, then this is the dream you need to pursue.

I want to give you an example of a goal you should *not* pursue. Imagine your goal is to be a famous singer. You might have a beautiful voice, but on the other hand you could have a "singing in the shower" type of voice. You know, the one that makes the neighbors' dogs howl. (That would be me!) If you are one of these people, I urge you to consider another dream. The reason is twofold. First, pursuing this type of dream would not beneficial to you or anyone else. Second, singing in the shower, out of tune, will never get you to celebrity status in the field of entertainment.

However, let me continue by saying that if the songs you are singing in the shower were written by you, then perhaps the goal you should pursue is to write music. Many famous composers cannot sing, but they write beautifully.

Now you have a list of dreams, two or three to start with, and you are passionate about them. These are the goals you should pursue. Begin by planning the execution of each dream.

Planning is a huge part of achieving your dreams. Maybe you don't like to work on the details, but you are great with the concepts. I completely understand. I'm that way, too. I really don't like to sit down and think of all the little steps I need to take in order to achieve my goals. But, honestly, this is the most necessary part of the process of moving forward and permanently changing your life. Without planning, you will dream and dream, but you will not produce results. In the end, you will be frustrated because you have not achieved anything. Ultimately, it will cause you to feel useless and worthless; you will doubt yourself and want to give up.

"A goal properly set is halfway reached." Zig ZIglar

Planning is half the battle. Honestly, once it's done you will feel incredible and invincible, and maintaining momentum will be much easier because your plan will remind you of the direction you want to go. Think of it this way: when you look at a picture every day, you are reminded of what the picture represents, but if you only see the picture once, the details will begin to fade and the intensity of the picture will diminish.

You can begin by asking yourself these questions and then add details to the answers[§]:

1. What material things will I need to accomplish my dream?

2. What education or licensing might I need that I do not currently have?

3. Who are the people and what organizations can help me achieve my goals?

4. What obstacles might I encounter during the process?

5. What are the first steps I need to take to start my journey?

Next, begin to answer each of these questions in detail. The more details you add, the more vivid your plan will be and the greater your chance of reaching your goals. Start with the first question and then move through each of the five questions. Write down the answers and add details. Each person will have a different way of completing the details.

---

§   A worksheet is included in the appendix titled "What I need to achieve my goals"

For example, I don't like writing down details, and it is easier for me to write just a few of them related to each question before moving on to the next question.

For example, one of my goals is to teach the information in this book to people live and online. I am passionate about sharing this message with everyone. I think about it all the time. I have thought about helping others my entire life. This work is my heart and soul. When I realized everything I had experienced was not only applicable to myself but to many others, I decided this was what I wanted to do.

I learned the process of reaching goals a couple of years earlier, and I had applied it to my life with great success, so I knew what to do. I sat down and started to answer the questions, but because I see the big picture and have trouble concentrating on the smaller details, I had a difficult time getting it all out of my head and written on paper.

I decided to write down the things that came to mind easily and then leave it; later, I would come back to it, maybe not until the next day. Then I would read it over and discover whether there were more details to write down. Writing this book was one of my dreams, and it came under the category of goals related to material things. This was an entirely new process that had to be detailed as a separate dream, but it was linked to my dream of teaching others how to heal themselves.

Whatever method you decide to use in order to answer these questions is completely up to you. The goal is to do it in as much detail as possible.

WHAT MATERIAL THINGS WILL YOU NEED TO ACCOMPLISH YOUR DREAM?

When achieving any goal, you will need certain things to help you. Let me give a simple example. If one of your dreams is to write a book, you will need to use certain material items. One item might be a writing pad and pen or pencil. Another item might be a computer with a word-processing program.

Think of all the material things you might need and write them down. Then you can go back and detail each item later. What type of writing pad will you use? Will it have lines or no lines? Do you want your pen to have blue or black ink? Which computer do you feel most comfortable with, and which word-processing program do you want to use?

It's perfectly okay if your list is not complete. Your plan will not be complete when you first start working on it, because there are things you may not be aware of when you start the process. Later, you might realize you need something different. The plan is going to change continuously, so think about as many things as you can and add them to your list as they come up. Remember to put as much detail in this as possible. The idea is to be able to visualize the items when you read your plan and make decisions about how to proceed.

WHAT OBSTACLES MIGHT YOU ENCOUNTER?

Inevitably, obstacles will arise on your path to overcoming your past. This is just a fact of life. God allows these obstacles. He chooses them to help you grow and become the person you need to be in order to realize your true purpose and reach your ultimate destiny. Romans 5:3-5 explains why we have obstacles in our life. "3 Not only so, but we also glory in our sufferings, because we know that suffering produces perseverance; 4 perseverance, character; and character, hope. 5 And hope does not put us to shame, because God's love has been poured out into our hearts through the Holy Spirit, who has been given to us." NIV

. . . .

"3 Not only so, but we also glory in our sufferings,
because we know that suffering produces perseverance;
4 perseverance, character; and character, hope. 5 And
hope does not put us to shame, because God's love has
been poured out into our hearts through the Holy Spirit,
who has been given to us." Romans 5:3-5 NIV

. . . .

You may have heard the story of Job in the Bible. If you have not heard this story you can read it in Book of Job. Here, I will give you a short version of Job's story.

Job was a wealthy man who was devoted to God and very faithful. He was well respected in his community, and he had a life that was desired by many. One day, Satan was going to and fro upon the Earth looking for someone to devour, when God said to him, "Have you considered my servant Job, for there is none like him in all the earth, a blameless and upright man who fears God and shuns evil?" (Job 1:8 NIV)

So Satan answered God, saying, "Does Job fear God for nothing? Have you not placed a hedge around him, around his household, and around all that he has on every side? You have blessed the work of his hands and his possessions have increased in the land." Job 1:9-10

Then Satan said to God that if he reached out his hand

and touched Job that he would curse Him. With this statement, God allowed Satan to have power over all Job had, but specifically he should not touch Job personally. So Satan began to wreak havoc on Job's businesses, family, and property. Job lost everything and was distraught. There were many other negative things that happened to Job but he never cursed God.

I did not understand that Satan had to first ask God for permission to present me with trouble and trials. I just thought I was a failure and that God didn't care about me. This was what I was told when I was a child. I believed I needed to be perfect before I could deserve to live without problems. How wrong could I have been? If you are thinking like this, you are wrong, too. Let me explain.

The end of the story of Job is that at the end of the trials and tribulations he encountered, he learned that he had too much pride in himself and his abilities. You see, God wants you to remember that you are wonderfully made, that you are a child of the King, and that all that you ask is yours if you just depend on Him and believe in Him.

Job believed in Him, but he had forgotten that everything he had achieved was because of God. When he realized this, he apologized and asked God for forgiveness. God gave Job back everything he had, plus even more than before. One consistency in this story is that Job never took his eyes away from the reason for his existence. He never cursed God, but held fast to the faithfulness he had for God. He could see there was a reason much higher than his present circumstance, and he chose to hold onto it, even when everyone around him was telling him he should curse God and die.

It does not matter who you are and what you might have done, where you have been or what you have been through, you can and will overcome your pain and suffering. One of the ways you can do this is to foresee as many obstacles as possible before they happen. You will not foresee all of them, but the more you anticipate ahead of time, the less time it will take to overcome them. You might even be able to avoid them completely.

Write every possible obstacle down on paper. It does not matter how large or how small, simply write it down. Then, for each one, begin to think about what will need to be done to prevent the obstacle or overcome it. For instance, if you have had problems in the past with drug or alcohol addictions, beginning the road to recovery can be difficult because so many in your life enabled you to use. Now that you are not using anymore you will be presented with the obstacle of your friends who are still using. They will likely want you to "hang out" with them. Of course, you can't do this because the temptation will be so great. So how will you overcome this situation? Will you just avoid them? See them only when they are sober or not high? Explain to them the reasons you don't want to be around them? Would it be reasonable to ask them to help you in your sobriety? Also, consider how you will make new friends who engage in more positive activities.

Write down all of the ways you might overcome this obstacle and then move on to the next. When you have your potential obstacles and solutions defined, you can move to the next step: determine what you personally need in order to achieve your goals. This does not have to be completed before adding answers to other questions. Just return to each question, adding more answers and details as you are able to think of them. This process can help you see the path to achieving your dream, so the more detail you include the better. You must keep moving forwards in the process. This concept cannot be emphasized enough.

WHAT DO YOU NEED?

As you begin to write down your obstacles, you may discover there are certain abilities or training you need to accomplish your goals. If this is the case, write them down and explain how you are going to get this additional training or ability. If you want to write a book, for example, you will need the ability to write. You can gain this ability with practice, so start by writing in a journal each day. This is a good practice, regardless of whether you want to write a book or not, because it can give you a good perspective about who you are, how you think, and your deepest desires. Journaling can even make you laugh when you read what you've written later. Consider taking an online writing class, and there are countless articles about how to write a book that can be downloaded for free on the Internet.

Perhaps you want to begin a new career, let's say in nursing, but you have no formal training. Obviously, you will need take classes and obtain the certification needed to enter this field. Write all of this down and begin to add the details as you discover them, so you will have a precise description of what is needed to achieve your new goals.

WHO DO YOU NEED TO HELP YOU?

Everyone needs help from someone. It doesn't matter if this is a life coach, a family member, a trusted friend, or a successful person in the field you are interested in. You need help and support. You cannot do it alone. I learned this the hard way. Perhaps you are so stubborn and independent you think you don't need help. I struggled for many years to overcome the vicious circle I was trapped in because I was too stubborn and proud to admit I had a problem and that I needed help. If this describes your attitude, you must immediately put aside your proud nature and ask someone for help. We were not designed to be totally independent. Even from the beginning of time when God created Adam, He said it was good but he saw that man needed a helper, so he created the beasts of the earth, the fish in the sea, and the birds of the air. Still, it was not enough, so he created Eve to be Adam's mate. You can find this story in the book of Genesis in the Bible.

. . . .

Then the Lord God said, "It is not good
for the man to be alone; I will make him a
helper suitable for him." Genesis 2:18

. . . .

Find someone to help you achieve your goals. Maybe it will be someone in business who has already done what you want to do. Don't be afraid to ask. Successful people are likely to feel honored if you ask them to mentor you and occasionally ask them questions about how they became a success. Perhaps you need moral support; find a local church and ask the members and the pastor for help. Get involved with local organizations that include people who have experienced the things you need to know. These organizations might include people in business and other professionals, parents, artists, and many others. If you want someone to help you, finding a group of like-minded people is important and usually easy.

Write down what you know you need and continue. This venture is a living, breathing experience that becomes alive when you put it into action. If you really and truly desire to improve your life, you will do whatever it takes to get there. My mentor, Zig Ziglar, often repeated speaker Joe Sabah's quote, "You don't have to be great to start, but you have to start to be great."

"You don't have to be great to start but you have to start to be great." Joe Sabah

WHAT IS THE NEXT STEP?

Now that you have the basic elements of your plan for achieving your goal, start dividing it into small steps. Do not worry about putting the steps in a specific order. Remember, your plan is not going to be 100 percent complete in the beginning. It lives and breathes along with you, so it is going to change as you discover more and redefine your goals and decisions.

Think of a small child – she only knows "this is mom" and "this is dad." But there is another person; at first, they are not sure yet who this person is; then later they learn it's their brother or sister. Soon, they discover how to walk, run, ride a bike, compete in sports or academics, and life continues to add more and more to their list of things they know.

You are like this child. As you continue through each day, you will be presented with experiences you don't totally understand, and it is up to you to learn from them. I was in my late thirties when I began to learn Spanish. I came from a small east Texas town where little Spanish was spoken, so I was never exposed to it. When I was in high school, we had the option to learn Spanish, but I did not see the need for it. Over 20 years later, I began to discover there was a world outside of my small East Texas town, and a large part of it spoke another language, Spanish or some other Latin-based language. I really did not think I would be able to learn it at such a late point in my life. Do you know the saying: "You can't teach an old dog new tricks?" It's not true. You really can, I know, because now I can read, write, and speak Spanish as a second language. My mom and my grandfather always told me I could do anything I wanted to do if I wanted it badly enough. This concept has helped me attain my goals, but it did not come without some hard lessons from lack of planning and foresight. This is what I am teaching, and I pray that you learn this valuable lesson from this chapter, because if you perform these steps in *any* area of your life you will succeed.

NOW WHAT?

This is quite possibly the easiest, yet hardest step of them all. It's easy because the answer is to simply start, but it's also hard because of personal doubt, lack of confidence, and fear of failure. I still experience these fears, but I am being as honest and as clear as I can at this moment. Fear is nothing more than False Evidence Appearing Real.

. . . .

God has not given us the spirit of fear but of power,
of love, and of a sound mind. 2 Timothy 1:7

. . . .

Take a look at the phrase "spirit of fear" from the 2 Timothy 1:7. Let me ask you, "What is a spirit?" Webster's Dictionary defines a spirit as: (1) an **animation of a vital principle** that is held to give life to a physical being, and (2) a **supernatural** being or essence. Looking at both definitions you can see they have one thing in common: spirit is not physical, but rather animation of a vital principle. It is an unreal characterization of a necessity. This animation, this supernatural being, gives life to the physical.

Now, knowing the thing you fear most is nothing more than an animation of your thoughts or past; laugh it off and take the first step. This step is usually the hardest; after it, the steps just get easier.

After you take that first step, even though it might feel scary, keep moving, building momentum, and ticking off each step. Add more steps, as needed, and delete those that are not needed. This is not a plan written in stone. You need to be somewhat flexible and open to suggestions. Remember you are not in this alone, because the people around you really want you to succeed.

There is an important concept here that needs to be emphasized. When you begin to take the steps in your plan, you are not only taking steps written on a piece of paper, you are designing your new future. Each step taken is a foundation that is being built to get you to the top. The first time I went to Mexico, my family took me to see the pyramids. They have always intrigued me because they are so precise in their structure, and they were built so many years ago without the assistance of technology to provide precision or equipment to form and place the stones. They were built to withstand time and the elements. How was this possible? It all started with a dream, developed into a plan, and was then executed, step by step, precisely, continuously, over a long period of time. Finally, these magnificent structures were created to fulfill the purpose and destiny of the men who conceived and built them.

Your life is like a pyramid. It begins with your dream, progresses into a plan, and is executed in fulfillment of your purpose. You are at the execution phase. Start with the first step and then move to the next. These steps, regardless of how small they may seem, are part of an integral structure that you can build by compounding each one, consistently, over time to create your ultimate success.

. . . .

"Every step you take going forward will help create a new you, a person you will not be ashamed of, a person you can feel good about, and when others see what you have done they will see you as a person to be admired." Janna Valencia

. . . .

Every step you take going forward will help create a new you, a person you will not be ashamed of, a person you can feel good about, and when others see what you have done they will see you as a person to be admired. They will look to you for help, just as you looked to others when you began this journey. It is time to continue to the next phase of your healing.

CHAPTER 8

Step 4: Your New World

Now that you are creating a new world to live in, it's time to share it with someone else. You don't have to stand on a stage and tell the world. You can make a difference right where you are, with the people you come into contact with every day.

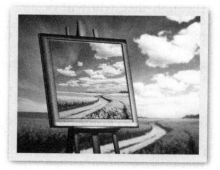

We are all born with a purpose. We walk through life trying to find purpose, as we explore different areas of our lives: professionally, educationally, personally, and almost always we are looking for purpose in our relationships with others, and using their lives as an example for our own. Looking to people who have achieved goals similar to ours, will help us reach find our true purpose.

Once you have identified your true destiny, prepare to take it to completion. Regardless of what means you are using, your destiny is to give others your wisdom and learning. Share your life and experience for the benefit of others.

Some people reach their ultimate destiny much faster than others. For those of us who did not find it until later in life, we look back wondering how we could have missed something so easily seen.

It is not important for you to accept my beliefs without question, but rather to understand the meaning of my words. Through this, you will be able to discover your true destiny and purpose. I am going to use personal experiences and stories from the most widely read book ever written, the Bible.

I was 50 years old before I found my purpose in life. I lived those 50 years experiencing many things along the way. I searched for my true destiny in school and didn't find it, although I did learn many subjects. I looked for it in other people and in relationships and didn't find it, but I learned much about how people think and what makes them do the things they do. I looked for my destiny through drug and alcohol abuse and found only pain and misery. From this, I learned that everyone has the ability to make good and bad decisions. I looked for it in work and my career, spending all of my working life dedicated to sales, management, and entrepreneurship, but I didn't find it there, either. However, I learned many things about business and that I loved helping others.

Once I realized that I liked helping others and I was naturally good at it, and had been for my entire life, I determined that my purpose and destiny was just this: to help others. Then the question became, "How?" I began looking, but I could not find the right avenue. I was always searching within my own world, through the things I had experienced and the places I knew. Through a series of events, I came to know about the family of Zig Ziglar, who was my mentor, and how his family was educating others to teach his message.

Something inside me wanted to be a part of this movement, so I made the decision to apply and was accepted. I attended the training, which is designed to walk you through each of the programs so you can experience what your eventual audience will experience when you teach them the same material. I was changed during that weeklong training. I finally saw my purpose and destiny. It was not in a job or a person or in a particular place; it was around me every day, wherever I was and whatever I was doing. It was the simple act of being myself and acting on the desires of my heart – please don't confuse this with every little whim, but overwhelming, burning desire. I learned how to be honest with every person I meet. Now I understand that my purpose is to "be the light" for others who have been hurt and carried their burdens for years, as they looked for their own purpose and destiny.

The Bible tells a story in John, Chapter 4, about Jesus. He was traveling and stopped to rest by a well near Samaria. A woman came to the well to draw water and Jesus asked her to give Him a drink. In those days, Jews did not have conversations with Samaritans so she was quite surprised.

The purpose of Jesus, when He was on Earth, was to make recompense for the sins of man by shedding His blood for our sins. In His time on the earth, He traveled, delivering the message and preparing others to deliver this message once He had ascended back in to the heavens with His Father, God. Knowing this, you will understand that when Jesus opened His mouth, the words He spoke were to teach of the life that was available through Him. So Jesus said to the woman that if she knew who He was, she would have asked *Him* for a drink. He went on to explain that the water He gives is "Living Water," and if we partake in it we will never thirst again because it will become a fountain of spiritual water inside of us.

He told the Samaritan woman intimate details about her personal life, which led her to believe He was a prophet. He went on to explain that the day was coming when all would worship God, the Father in spirit and in truth. The woman said she knew the Messiah was coming and that He would tell the truth in all things. At this point, Jesus told her that He was the One who had been prophesied to come.

Wherever Jesus went, he told stories like this. He performed signs and wonders; He told people the way to everlasting life and explained to them how to live on the earth. He taught people right from wrong. His very life is an example for us to follow.

We do not need special training or education to live our destiny. We only have to live as we are, as an example of what is good and right. The rest will come to us. Every person's purpose is to be an example for those whom he has the privilege to meet. We should not desire to be something we are not, only to be the best of who we already are.

I have tried to be many things I am not. In high school, I wanted to be part of the "popular" crowd, so I tried out for the cheerleading team. While performing a simple jump, I fell and embarrassed myself, simply because I was trying to be someone I was not. Now, I understand that the status we attribute to others is irrelevant, and that we are all given talents based on who we really are, not whom we think we should be. Paul explains this in 1 Corinthians 7: 17 "Nevertheless, each person should live as a believer in whatever situation the Lord has assigned to them, just as God has called them. This is the rule I lay down in all the churches." NIV

"Nevertheless, each person should live as a believer in whatever situation the Lord has assigned to them, just as God has called them. This is the rule I lay down in all the churches." 1 Corinthians 7:17

The experiences I have been through in my life are not different from those you might have experienced. Only the details are different. These experiences are meant to build character, strength, and knowledge for the journey to our destiny. They also teach us how to help others find their true purpose.

Many of us go through life fighting our destiny. Let me explain. The experience I had in high school is a good example. I was not made to be a cheerleader for the football team, but I was made to be a cheerleader of life. If I had seen it then, my life experiences would have been quite different. I was a leader and a coach, and the people I made contact with always looked to me for support and encouragement. You, too, have wonderful qualities. If you were the smart kid in class, people always looked to you for guidance. If you participated in sports and were the "star" of the team, people looked to you for strength and inspiration.

We are all examples for each other in some way. It's our responsibility to use our gifts and serve as examples that will encourage others. However, people who don't have a purpose sometimes misconstrue this. They try to find purpose, but they end up becoming something they are not. They go through life getting training to do something they really don't want to do because of the status it holds, or because someone else wants it for them. Really, all we need to do is to be ourselves and use our gifts as an example to help someone else. Colossians, Chapter 3, explains that if we stop doing things that do not encourage and edify, and we do the things that will – while being thankful for all we have, whether it is little or much – we will be contented. This is such a simple statement, but it is profound. All we need do is accept what we have and who we are, right now.

Throughout life, we are presented with opportunities to discover our destiny. If we take advantage of these opportunities, we will have deeper understanding and our path will become ever more clear. Our individual purpose will begin to reveal itself. However, other opportunities will also arise demanding that we make decisions. These other opportunities, can take us down paths that might be misleading; a potential detour might occur and prevent us from achieving our purpose. Some might call this "making bad choices," but I believe that in the midst of the choices we make there are events and individuals who can lead us in the right direction, and those that will lead us in the wrong direction. As you continue taking the steps leading to your true purpose, these other events and individuals might guide or distract you, but most often they do not know what effects they are causing in the spiritual world. They truly think they are helping you.

I made many wrong decisions and travelled down many wrong paths that were merely detours. Some of the choices I made were simply bad ones, but sometimes it was not so apparent. On the outside, they looked like good choices that would bring great returns and happiness, but if I had listened to the small voice inside that was telling me something was not my heart's desire, that it really in my best interests, I would have made a different choice, a better choice.

When an opportunity presents itself in the form of an event or a person and you are required to make a decision, ask yourself: "Will this take me closer to or further away from where I want to be, what I want to do, or who I want to be? Is this potential opportunity for my higher good?"

When an opportunity presents itself in the form of an event or a person and you are required to make a decision, ask yourself: "Will this take me closer to or further away from where I want to be, what I want to do, or who I want to be?" Janna Valencia

These questions will remind you to pause and think about the possible outcome before you make a decision. Additionally, if you have used the plan outlined in previous chapters, you already have complete awareness of your path and your goals.

To make the best choices, you need to be informed. In the past, when I made bad choices and took the wrong roads, I was not informed. I was learning in defense, not in offense. What I mean by this is that I would make an uninformed choice, and then learn it was a bad choice *after* I experienced the results. If I had taken the time to listen and to seek out better options when I was presented with the choices, I might have chosen differently. Ultimately, I would have come to know my purpose much sooner.

It does not matter what stage of life you are in, you can still find your purpose and live your destiny. It does not matter how old you are, but rather the strength of your desire to achieve your goals. You can achieve your destiny if you are determined to take the appropriate steps to get there.

We are all destined to bring hope, inspiration, strength, and love to others. We are the light, where there was only darkness. We do this by being present in truth, honesty, humility, charity, and love. If you have never experienced this, it's time for it. This will open a door for you to experience your true purpose and live your destiny. The way to enter this door is to knock.

Ask, and it will be given to you, seek, and you will find, knock, and it will be opened to you. Matthew 7:7

In the end, or the beginning, we find our purpose in being an example for others, just as Jesus did for the disciples and they did for others. 1 Corinthians 12 explains that you have been given certain abilities to help you serve as an example, so start to use them. There is no need to look any further; you already possess everything you need. Search within yourself and find the things that make your heart beat faster, that give you chill bumps when you think about them, and that you can see when you close your eyes. These are your gifts. Use them for all that is good.

For God so loved the world that he gave His only Son, and that whoever believes in Him, should not perish but have everlasting life. John 3:16

So begin to take the truth to everyone you know. Be the light for someone who has none, give inspiration where there is hopelessness, and be an example for those who are on a self-destructive path. Pray that they find their way back and discover their purpose.

Give and it will be given to you. Luke 6:38 NIV

It is your world and it is yours to make it what you want it to be. In the words of Zig Ziglar: "You can have everything you want in life if you will just help enough other people get what they want."

CHAPTER 9

Step 5: Unconditional Love

Unconditional love is an important and deep subject. First, let's look at what the words actually mean. The word "unconditional" is defined in Webster's Dictionary as being "without conditions or limits." It's described for people learning English as, "not limited in any way, complete or absolute."

"Love" is defined as a feeling of strong and constant affection. So, it seems unconditional love is a strong constant feeling of affection that knows no limitations and is always accepting.

Have you ever felt love that was truly unlimited? You

might say, "Yes" without first thinking about it, but stop and consider this concept of love. Unconditional love means you could still love the person who beat you until you were almost dead, or the husband or wife who cheated on you with another person. Now this is another story, or is it?

The last time I experienced betrayal, I was in a different frame of mind. Instead of just giving in to the same pain, I stood up and did something different. I began processing it the same way I had always done, but because of the new insights I had gained with the Ziglar Certification training, I knew that if I continued processing it the same way as in the past, I would be destined to continue creating the same scenario with yet another man. Of course, I didn't want this to happen, so I decided to change my behavior. This time, I accepted my husband's infidelity. Then, I forgave him. Why? There are two reasons.

. . . .

For if ye forgive men their trespasses, your heavenly Father will also forgive you. Matthew 6:14 KJV

. . . .

First, I forgave him because I was told to forgive, just as my Savior forgives us all. I knew that by forgiving others I would also be forgiven.

Second, I had recently been studying why people have certain types of problems in their life, particularly in marriage. I learned that when you enter into marriage with unresolved pain and hurt from the past, it results in an inability to have a healthy relationship.

Sometimes we have to go through difficult circumstances more than once to find the truth and overcome them. This is what happened to me. When I finally realized that I had entered into another relationship under unhealthy pretenses, and he had been unfaithful because of similar problems in his past, I could not leave the relationship without forgiving him.

I turned to God, the fountain of unconditional love. Through His support, I was able to forgive my husband and myself. Then the oddest thing happened. It was not at all odd when you know how unconditional love works, but at that point it seemed odd. I looked at this man, my husband, through different eyes. Even in the midst of all that had happened, I held no ill will against him. I understood his pain; I accepted that our relationship had been founded on negative pretenses; and I put everything in the hands of God. Then, I was able to love him unconditionally.

*For all have sinned, and fall short of the
glory of God. Romans 3:23*

I know you must be thinking I'm crazy, but I truly loved
him. It was not the passionate love of a man and woman or
the warm tingly feeling of new lovers. It was a love that sur-
passed human understanding; it was not because of anything
he had done or said. It was because he, too, is a Child of God.
He experienced pain in his life that was different than mine,
and he had no idea what was happening to him, or why. Now,
he is in the beginning stages of learning and making his way
through the same steps I have been taking.

In order to love unconditionally, you must understand the
events in your past completely and how they have affected
your life. You must also understand there are reasons why you
were hurt. Just as there are reasons to experience hurt in your
life, the other person has also experienced pain. Someone
once said, "two wrongs don't make a right." They are correct.
You must be able to humble yourself and say, "Okay, I get it!"
I will forgive and I will love.

Jesus is a perfect example of unconditional love. We condemned Him to die a horrible death. We hung Him on a

cross after He had been beaten so badly that His body was disfigured, His hands and feet were nailed to the cross. After all that, He still forgave us and loved us. He said it with His own lips before He died.

. . . .

Father forgive them for they know not
what they do. Luke 23:34 NIV

. . . .

I want to be clear about this because it's important. I am not telling you that you should love what has happened to you. Jesus was in excruciating pain from what had been done to Him. When he asked God to forgive us, it was not that He forgave us for the act, but for not knowing we were doing something terrible when we crucified the Son of God. When you read the verse again, you will notice that is says "because they *know not* what they do."

Jesus continued to love us because although we knew what we were doing, we did not know why. Yes, I continued to love my husband after he abused me. This does not mean I should have permitted the abuse, but now I am able to love him unconditionally because he did not (and does not) understand why he treated me so badly.

There is another saying that is not direct scripture from

the bible, but it is based in scripture (Jude 1:22-23). "Love the sinner, hate the sin." This really sums it all up.

Loving unconditionally comes with the responsibility to speak the truth. Now, this does not mean that you can just open your mouth and let all of the "stuff" come out. You need to take care. Remember when you were a teenager and you got to use the car for the first time? Perhaps it was your parents who let you use it, or maybe a friend, but what was the one thing you remember them telling before you took it? "Be careful." This meant look both ways before you hit the gas, don't speed, stop at all signs and lights, no racing, buckle up, use turn signals, park away from other cars, and watch the other drivers, because they are unpredictable.

These two simple words had a lot of meaning. They did not need explanation; you knew that they meant. In the same way, we should speak the truth with love when we are telling someone how he or she has hurt us. It should not be done in anger, and it should not be filled with blaming details from the past.

When you are hurt and angry, you might lash out in an attempt to make someone else feel what you have felt. You might say things that are hurtful and cause pain. I did this in all of my relationships. Something would happen to hurt me and I would lash out against the other person with words that caused more suffering. Even if they were true, there is a right and wrong way to speak. I always chose the wrong way. That is, until this last time. During the relationship, I was guilty of lashing out. I had to apologize for this. When I finally got the opportunity to talk to him about what had happened between us, I was able to explain it to him calmly, instead of saying ugly things to cause pain. Being hurt by someone does not give you the right to hurt the person back, as much as you might want to believe it does. In Romans 12:19, God says that vengeance is His. This means that He will take care of the wrong that has been done to you. Throughout the Bible, there are stories of God's vengeance. I do not want any of this in my life, and I feel for anyone who has to bear it.

The point is, when you tell someone about the hurt they have caused you simply state you feel hurt and forgive them. Allow your new understanding about the past to fill your heart, mind and soul, and you will be able to love others unconditionally.

CHAPTER 10

The Power of Your Mind

The day is coming when you will look back on your life and wonder why you wasted so much time on trivial things, put so much emphasis on them, and allowed them to consume your life.

When I was a teenager, I would sit at my grandmother's kitchen bar watching her cook and listening to her tell stories about her life, the latest things that happened to her or around her, or complaining about something my grandfather said or did, which was always something! One thing, in particular, I remember is that she worried about everything. I would ask myself, "Why does she worry so much?" I never wanted to be like her. Afterwards, I watched my mother become my grandmother, also worrying about so many things. Not so long ago, I found myself worrying, too.

We worry as we become older because we are more aware of what can go wrong; we put too much attention on everything that's wrong in the world. Most of what we hear on the news is about death and destruction, and we worry about our own demise. Perhaps we should remain as we were in our youth, ignorant of worldly events.

We watch movies about Superman, Batman, Spiderman, and other super-human heroes fight the battle against evil. We also watch movies about death and destruction, drug dealers, murderers, and thieves. What an imagination humans have to be able to create these movies.

Our minds can generate creative ideas with such force that they become reality. We have been given gifts that are akin to being super-human. I'm not talking about leaping over the highest buildings or swinging from building to building from webs that project from our wrists. The super-human abilities we have are mental, and tapping into this inner power and developing our ideas can produce great results.

Everything you take into your body, mind, or spirit and let digest becomes part of you. This is true with food, the words you speak, and the things you hear, see, and experience. If everything around you is negative, you will be negative; if your environment is positive, you will be positive. Constant exposure to either will affect your life proportionally.

. . . .

"You are who you are and what you are because of what has gone into your mind. You can change who you are and what you are by changing what goes into your mind." Zig Ziglar

. . . .

Remember when you were young? You didn't know you couldn't do certain things, although you had dreams of being great. Perhaps you dreamed of being a President, doctor, lawyer, or movie star. It was not until you were told that you could not do something that you began to put limitations on yourself. When you first tried to ride a bicycle, you failed many times before you finally achieved success, but you didn't stop trying because no one told you that you couldn't do it. Actually, it was quite the opposite; they encouraged you to keep trying. It's the same with any endeavor you have ever ventured into. If you are encouraged, you will make the effort. If you are discouraged, you will not.

Don't put limitations on yourself. Believe that you can attain your desires, work toward them and you can make it happen.

. . . .

"I've failed over and over and over again in my life and that is why I succeed. I can accept failure, everyone fails at something. But I can't accept not trying. Some people want it to happen, some wish it would happen, others make it happen." Michael Jordan

. . . .

In the Bible, the Book of Joshua, Chapter 14, Caleb, at 85 years old, is living an ageless life. He comes upon the mountain of Hebron, where he encounters the Anakim, who were giants and very strong warriors.

Caleb said, "Today I am as strong as when I entered the service, when I was 40 years old." He *believed* that he was as strong at 85 as he was when he was 40. He entered into war with the giants and defeated them, taking the mountain as his own. It was the power of Caleb's mind that kept him strong.

We have many experiences in life, some of which bring us much joy and happiness. Others might be painful and bring sadness. Regardless of the experience, our mind processes it, and it becomes part of us. This will have an effect on how we make decisions in the future. These experiences help us become more intelligent; they will lead us to or away from our destiny.

All of the experiences we have, good and bad, are beneficial. None of them can keep us from our destiny if we choose to use them in a beneficial way. Allowing negative experiences to become internalized can cause us to make decisions about our future based on fear and weakness. Instead, if we digest our negative experiences as life lessons and use them in balance with positive outcomes, we can make decisions made from a position of strength rather than weakness. You have heard me say this in previous chapters but I want you to hear me.

How many failures did Einstein have before he finally realized his destiny and used his knowledge to become one of the most brilliant men of all time? He struggled in school and dropped out; he had speech problems and was known as a "draft dodger." If he had never experienced these things, he might not have achieved anything. Even more importantly, if he had let what happened to him in his youth stop him from continuing his path to achieving his destiny, we might have never even known his name.

You might be thinking it's easy for me to say this, but it's something else to actually do it. You're right. It's very easy to say something, but to follow through can be a challenge. Once you have made a commitment to your purpose, the sky could fall around you and you will continue moving towards your destiny. You may pause to get a better understanding of what you have just experienced, but you will not stop. You have a fire burning inside you that keeps you up at night and wakes you up early; it drives you to keep moving forward even when the world considers your situation as a catastrophe.

By now, you know your purpose. Commit to it, and let it become part of you. Eat it, drink it, live it, and when the rain comes and the winds blow you will not be shaken. The power that you hold in your mind has the ability to take you far beyond what you could ever imagine if you use it the way it was designed. Your brain is a magnificent, mysterious piece of matter that is only limited by your imagination. It's insane, but true, that you will likely limit it over and over again before something in you clicks and you open the roadblock and allow your mind to conceive the thing you have not been able to recognize. Once you remove this roadblock, you will begin to fully achieve your dreams. Your level of perseverance in achieving your goals will determine your success.

The Road to Healing is a discovery process. The longer

you travel it, the more revelations you will have. You will become stronger, smarter, happier, healthier, prosperous, and you will know, beyond all doubt, that you are walking in harmony with your destiny.

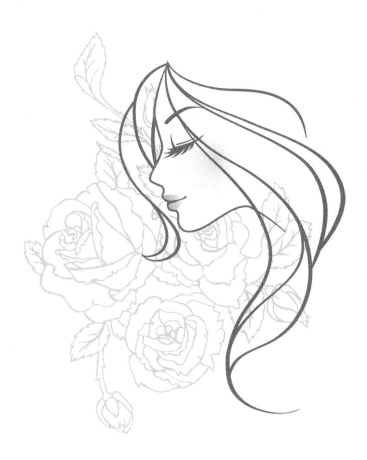

About the Author

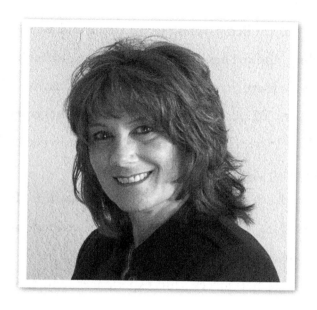

Janna Valencia was raised on a farm in a small east Texas town, where she learned good Christian values and hard work. She experienced many aspects of life, both good and bad, learning valuable lessons in life. She became a wife and mother at 19. She is a survivor of physical and mental abuse and drug addiction. She experienced the betrayal of sexual addictions in her marriages—and she received her victory when she received Jesus Christ as her personal Savior and began to live again.

Janna has studied psychology and drug and alcohol abuse counseling, and she has used this education and her life experiences to achieve personal success and help others.

She spent 25 years in retail sales and management, and more than 15 years as a successful business owner and avid entrepreneur.

Today she is a born again Christian, author, Robbins Madanes Life Coach, Ziglar Legacy Certified Speaker/ Trainer, and business consultant.

Janna uses her success, life experiences, and training to show others how they, too, can live a victorious, whole, and fulfilling life. She teaches individuals and groups in person, by phone, and via webinars. Janna conducts live events, where she teaches the information in the *Road to Healing* with hands-on activities and participation from attendees. She has established an online study program, Victory Academy, which allows students to experience the Road to Healing at their own pace, using videos to aid in the process.

Her business programs are taught live, on site. During these programs, she conducts in depth interviews with the owners and employees to develop and implement the needed structure and systems to move their business into growth, efficiency, and the real reason a person owns a business: freedom – freedom to have more time to spend with family, earn more money, take vacations, and live with less demands and more benefits. Yes, you can have all that!

Janna has been commissioned by God to preach the gospel, delivering the Good News to audiences around the world. Her life experiences and her salvation are testimony that anyone can overcome their past and live a happy, full life. She has been led by God to deliver her message without charge and only asks for her sponsors to prayerfully consider a donation.

"She opens her mouth in wisdom and the teaching of kindness is on her tongue." Proverbs 31:26

To learn more about Janna Valencia, her coaching, business consulting, ministry, speaking, and training, or to purchase her online study programs, books, audios, or videos, please visit www.JannaValencia.com.

About Julie Ziglar Norman

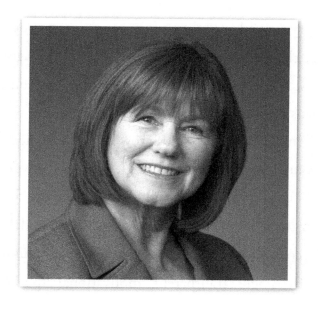

Julie Ziglar was her father's editor for almost 20 years, and she is a winner of the coveted Guideposts Writers Workshop contest. She is also a past president of the Texas Herpetological Society and the 2009 recipient of the Journey of Sisters, Honorary Sister Award.

Her background in sales, business management, and the

service industry, as well as her experience as a wife, single mother, step-parent, grandmother, and widow, enable her to relate well to just about everyone! Julie's riveting presentation style and her ability to create an internal desire for positive change have contributed to her being recognized as the most meaningful female motivator speaking on public platforms today.

Julie lives in the sleepy little town of Alvord, Texas with one rescued cat, two rescued dogs, and one "on purpose" horse. She and her late husband Jim Norman have four children, thirteen grandchildren, and three great-grandchildren.

Julie continues her father's legacy as a dynamic, disarming, and refreshingly transparent motivational speaker and author. She is comfortable speaking to a small group of 25 or a venue of 25,000. Her unique experience of being raised by the "motivators' motivator" has given her a perspective on life and work that keeps her audiences laughing, crying, and taking notes.

Carrying her father's legacy of encouragement into the next generation is an honor and a privilege that Julie never expected or sought, but her willingness to accept the challenge has already inspired over a million people in America and abroad. Her vibrant style of delivery, her honest and transparent assessment of life, and her willingness to share intimate details of personal failures, as well as personal triumphs, has made her a popular crowd favorite.

As her famous father once did, Julie has shared the platform with great leaders, including General Colin Powell, Rudy Giuliani, President George W. Bush, Laura Bush, Howard Putnam, Lou Holtz, Steve Forbes, Sarah Palin, and many others. She has delivered keynotes for corporations, direct sales organizations, annual association conventions, not-for-profit organizations and ministries, women's organizations, and entrepreneurial groups.

To learn more about Julie Ziglar Norman and her speaking and training, or if you are interested in having Julie speak at one of your events, please visit **www.JulieZiglarNorman.com**

About Zig Ziglar

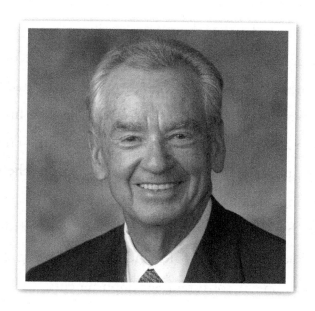

Affected at a very early age by the death of his father, Zig Ziglar learned firsthand the importance of self-reliance and a balanced work ethic. This foundation would eventually become his motto: "You can have everything in life you want if you will just help enough other people get what they want."

Recognized by his peers as the quintessential motivational genius of our times, Zig Ziglar's unique delivery style and powerful messages have earned him many honors. Today he is considered one of the most versatile authorities on the science of human potential. As a patriot, he was recognized three times in the Congressional Record of the United States for his work with youth in the drug war and for his dedication to America and the free enterprise system. Titans of business, politics, and sports consider him to be the single greatest influence in their lives.

From his humble beginnings in Yazoo City, Mississippi, to the Hall of Fame in Sales and Marketing, Zig Ziglar's career was one of consistent accomplishments. The earliest victories in large national sales organizations and a professional speaking career that allowed him to traverse this globe are the foundation upon which the corporation that bears his name is built. In July 2001, the National Speakers Association honored Zig Ziglar with their highest award, "The Cavett."

Since 1970, individuals and institutions have utilized an extensive collection of Ziglar audios, videos, books, and training curriculum. The client list of Ziglar, Inc., reads like a "Who's Who" in American and global business. Ten of his

33 books have been on the bestseller lists, and his titles have been translated into more than 40 languages and dialects.

Though he died in November of 2012, Zig Ziglar is still rated by his peers, as well as by audiences everywhere, as one of the best and most versatile motivational speakers, teacher and trainer to ever live. He traveled the world over, delivering his messages of humor, hope, and enthusiasm to audiences of all kinds and sizes.

Besides the books he has written, Zig Ziglar's practical, tri-dimensional philosophy has been incorporated into an extensive array of audio, video, and printed training tools, in addition to seminars and workshops.

Zig was happily "over-married" to his wife of 66 years, Jean, whom he lovingly called "Sugar Baby" in the privacy of their home. When speaking of her publically he called her "the Redhead!" He was a committed family man, a dedicated patriot, and an active church member. He was chosen by the Mississippi Broadcasting Association as "Mississippian of the Year" in 1985 and as "Communicator of the Year" by the Sales and Marketing Executives International in 1991. In April of 1995, he received his Honorary Doctor of Humanities from Oklahoma Christian University of Science and Arts, and was named an Ambassador of Free Enterprise by Sales & Marketing Executives International Academy of Achievement. He was recognized as one of the Toastmasters International Five Outstanding Speakers of 1997 for Contributions to the Art of Public Speaking, and in 1998 he received the Sales and Marketing Executives Leadership Award and an Honorary Doctor of Letters Degree for Contribution to Literature on Human Potential from Southern Nazarene University. In August 1999, he received the National Speakers Association Master of Influence Award and the Toastmasters International Golden Gavel Award. In 2001, he was selected to receive the Cavett Award, the National Speakers Association's most cherished award, presented annually to the member whose accomplishments over the years have reflected outstanding credit, respect, honor, and admiration in the Association and speaking profession.

To learn more about Zig Ziglar, the Ziglar Legacy Training Program, Ziglar events, or to purchase any of Zig Ziglar's bestselling books, audios, or DVDs please visit www.ziglarcertified.com/jannavalencia

About Joyce Meyer

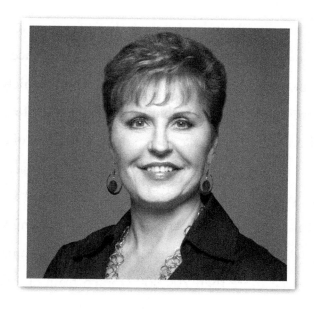

Joyce Meyer is one of the world's leading practical Bible teachers. A *New York Times* bestselling author, her books have helped millions of people find hope and restoration through Jesus Christ. Through *Joyce Meyer Ministries*, she teaches on a number of topics with a particular focus on the mind, mouth, moods, and attitudes. Her candid communication style allows her to share openly and practically about her experiences so others can apply what she has learned to their lives.

Joyce hosts a TV and radio show, *Enjoying Everyday Life*, which broadcasts worldwide to a potential audience of 4.5 billion people. She has authored 100 books, which have been translated into more than 100 languages. More than 12 million of her books have been distributed free of charge around the world, and each year millions of copies are sold.

Joyce conducts close to a dozen domestic and international conferences every year, teaching people to enjoy their everyday lives. For 30 years, her annual women's conference has attracted more than 200,000 women from all over the world to St. Louis for specifically themed teachings by her and guest speakers.

Through her teachings, God has provided opportunities to meet the needs of the suffering and bring the Gospel in a practical way. Joyce's passion to help hurting people is foundational to the vision of *Hand of Hope*, the mission's arm of *Joyce Meyer Ministries*. These outreaches around the globe include feeding programs, medical care, homes for orphans, and programs combating human trafficking. In her hometown of St. Louis, Joyce and Dave, her husband, founded the St. Louis Dream Center (SLDC) in 2000. The SLDC serves the inner city through hands-on programs targeted at reaching the lost and hurting with the love of Christ.

Over the years, God has provided Joyce with many opportunities to share her testimony and the life-changing message of the Gospel. Having suffered sexual abuse throughout her childhood, as well as just dealing with the struggles of everyday life, Joyce discovered the freedom to live victoriously by applying God's Word to her life and, in turn, she strives to help others do the same.

Joyce is, and continues to be, an incredible testimony of the dynamic, redeeming work of Jesus Christ.

To learn more about Joyce Meyer, her ministry, engagements, events, to purchase her bestselling books, audios, and videos, or to donate to her ministry and help reach the world with the Good News of Jesus Christ and His gift of eternal life, visit **www.joycemeyer.org**.

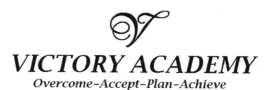

VICTORY ACADEMY
Overcome–Accept–Plan–Achieve

Now there is a way to interactively learn how to walk the Road to Healing. Janna created Victory Academy as an additional source to discover your limiting beliefs, walk you through the steps to overcome them, plan your future and achieve your destiny. This online course included hours of video, worksheets and course material that you have access to for life.

It has never been easier to listen and learn how to overcome what holds you back and achieve your true destiny.

As a way to say thank you for purchasing Road to Healing, Janna is offering you a special discount on Victory Academy. The normal price of the basic course is $149.00. When you use your special code RTH1 you will receive a $50.00 discount on the price.

Purchase the premium package which includes the course and a one hour consultation with Janna to help you gain focus and clarity in the process and you will get a discount of $75.00 off of the regular price of 349.99. Use discount code RTH2

If you would like to purchase the platinum subscription package, it includes the Victory Academy online course, a private coaching session with Janna each month and access to all live group calls in addition to an invitation for two to attend a live Victory is Yours event. The regular monthly price for the subscription is $149.00. Use the code RTHVIP1 and receive a monthly discount of $50.00

"You can achieve everything in life that you want. Let me show you how." Janna Valencia

APPENDIX

DREAM SHEET

Write all of your dream on this page.

DREAM SHEET

Write all of your dream on this page.

CATEGORIZE YOUR DREAMS

Each dream falls into one of these areas of your life.

Write the dream in the appropriate category.

Family

Personal

Mental

Spiritual

Professional

Health

Financial

MY WHY

Write all of the compelling, passionate reasons why you want to achieve your goals on this page.

MY WHY

*Write all of the compelling, passionate reasons why you want
to achieve your goals on this page.*

WHAT I NEED TO ACHIEVE MY GOALS

What material things will I need to accomplish my dream?
What education or licensing might I need that I do not
currently have?

WHAT I NEED TO ACHIEVE MY GOALS

Who are the people and what organizations can help me achieve my goals?
What obstacles might I encounter during the process?
What are the first steps I need to take to start my journey?

JOURNAL OF MY PROGRESS

JOURNAL OF MY PROGRESS

JOURNAL OF MY PROGRESS

JOURNAL OF MY PROGRESS

JOURNAL OF MY PROGRESS

JOURNAL OF MY PROGRESS

JOURNAL OF MY PROGRESS

JOURNAL OF MY PROGRESS

JOURNAL OF MY PROGRESS

JOURNAL OF MY PROGRESS

Made in the USA
Middletown, DE
14 September 2023

38497677R00099